- The drug that makes you young again—*or does it?*

- Oxygen starvation, free radicals, sludging and "clinkers"—*hidden culprits* in senility.

- Vitamins that have *restored* the "hopelessly senile" to good health.

- *Junk foods* and their role in promoting senility.

- Safe—and *vitally necessary exercise*—for the aging.

- Complete information on *needed nutrients* and their food sources.

> In a book about the causes and cure of senility— that combines practical, easy-to-follow recommendations with remarkable case histories and a fascinating account of medical "detective work"—two authorities on the subject present a progam for enjoying old age—*not dreading it!*

Other Keats Books of Relevant Interest

Brain Allergies: The Psycho-Nutrient Connection
by William H. Philpott, M.D. and Dwight K. Kalita, Ph.D.

The Complete Vitamin E Book
by Wilfrid E. Shute, M.D.

Diet and Disease
by E. Cheraskin, M.D., W.M., Ringsdorf, D.M.D.,
and J.D. Clark, D.D.S.

The Heart and Vitamin E
by Evan V. Shute, M.D.

Mental and Elemental Nutrients
by Carl C. Pfeiffer, M.D., Ph.D.

Orthomolecular Nutrition
by Abram Hoffer, M.D., Ph.D. and Morton Walker, D.P.M.

Physician's Handbook on Orthomolecular Medicine
edited by Roger J. Williams, Ph.D., and Dwight K. Kalita, Ph.D.

The Saccharine Disease
by T.L. Cleave, M.D.

NUTRIENTS TO AGE WITHOUT SENILITY

ABRAM HOFFER, M.D., PH.D.
and MORTON WALKER, D.P.M.

Introduction by
ROGER J. WILLIAMS, PH.D.

Keats Publishing, Inc. ■ New Canaan, Connecticut

NUTRIENTS TO AGE WITHOUT SENILITY

ISBN: (hardcover) 0-87983-217-7
          (paperback) 0-87983-218-5

Library of Congress Catalog Number 79-93428

Printed in the United States of America

Keats Publishing, Inc.
36 Grove Street, New Canaan, Connecticut 06840

DEDICATED TO

CLARA HOFFER, my mother, who first alerted me to the
value of vitamin B-3 in reversing senile changes
and
RAE WALKER, my mother, who is lively and alert, busy
with living, and sharing herself with others.

CONTENTS

INTRODUCTION

THE PROBLEM of aging and senility is of almost universal interest among adults. In this book on *Nutrients to Age Without Senility*, Abram Hoffer, M.D., Ph.D. and Morton Walker, D.P.M., present a large body of valuable information which potentially can help everybody slow down the inevitable aging process and prevent the unnecessary senile syndrome.

In the Huxley Institute sponsored National Conference in 1972 on Health Care for the Aging, I called attention to the fact that statistical "man," as he ages, may have a slight impairment of hearing, some balding, a little greying of hair, reduced vision, the loss of some teeth, a lessening of heart function, a slight loss of agility, a blunting of memory, a slight loss of sex urge, an increase in imbalance, and a few other changes.

Dr. Hoffer and Dr. Walker, however, in this book, are obviously not interested in statistical "man." They are interested in the aging of *real* people. They are concerned with you and me. Their discussions reveal a full appreciation of how different aspects of getting old become real problems in actual life. The two doctors treat the topics of aging and senility in a comprehensive way. Anyone who is interested in his or her own welfare during the aging process should read and try to digest the contents of this book and put them to work for his or her benefit.

From my personal experience in passing part way through the aging process, I enthusiastically endorse the idea that

1

by providing yourself with *all* the needed nutrients, exercising adequately, and avoiding environmental poisons, it is possible to do marvelous things for one's entire self. This book does not deal with trifling concerns!

Ideally, toward the end of life we should fall apart all at once and be gone like Oliver Wendell Holmes's "wonderful one-hoss shay." Drs. Hoffer and Walker have written a book which should help everyone in his or her approach to this ideal. As they make clear, every kind of essential nutrient comes into play in the promotion and prolongation of healthy life. It is a program of living that is worthwhile to follow.

—ROGER J. WILLIAMS, Ph.D.
June, 1980

PREFACE

FOLLOWING many years of clinical experience, I have concluded that senility can, in most cases, be prevented or treated and that chronic nutritional deficiencies play a large role in causing this disease. With Morton Walker, I decided to present the results of our experience which we gained from studying the medical literature and from our own observations.

Dr. Walker and I hope we can dissuade our readers away from the sterile view that senility inevitably accompanies aging. Enough is known to prove that senility is preventable. Each one of us alive who does not avoid senility is simply showing ignorance of the biological factors which allow its onset.

We will present the facts and hypotheses about aging and senility to allow anyone interested in living out life in full possession of his or her mental faculties to do so—or at least to try. But our program must begin as early as possible; the closer one is to senility, the more difficult it is to prevent it.

Our conviction is based upon two kinds of evidence: the first is the accumulated observations made by our predecessors and contemporaries in medicine, science, nutrition, and the second by non-professional observers, which have been recorded. There are references at the end of each chapter which document in the text the reports of a few scientists who have been pioneers in observing and in creating hypotheses about the process of aging.

The second kind of evidence is direct, such as is preferred in a court of law. From 1954, when I first realized what improved nutrition could do in reversing and preventing senility, I have observed similar beneficial effects in a number of my elderly patients. Within my immediate family, no one has become senile in the past twenty-five years, even though two had begun to show evidence of senility before they were started on nicotinic acid.

In Chapter One, we have outlined the evidence for our conclusions that senility is not inevitable, even if the first symptoms have occurred, while in Chapters Two and Three, we have described the aging changes which gradually occur from the stresses of our industrialized society. Chapter Four contains a discussion of the modern hypotheses to explain the aging process. Being hypotheses, these chapters are not carved in stone and probably will be markedly altered as new information accrues.

The next two chapters outline why we have concluded that senility is a form of chronic malnutrition; whenever I see a senile man or woman, I visualize the many decades of malnutrition which preceded this unhappy condition. We blame the heavy consumption of food artifact—junk food. We believe there will be a steady increase in the incidence of senility in industrialized countries, since the swing toward food artifact has not been halted. It is estimated that in a few years as much food will be sold in restaurants and fast food outlets as in supermarkets.

In Chapters Seven and Eight, we describe the vitamins and minerals which appear to be implicated most directly. But good food is not enough; exercise or physical fitness is equally important and we discuss this in Chapter Nine. The last chapter is an outline of a vitamin-containing substance used in reversing senile changes. The vitamin is para amino-benzoic acid, and the compound is known as GH3 or Gerovital. It is a special solution of procaine. Over the years, public pressure and demand have made this

European discovery more acceptable. Recent studies have confirmed the claims made for it.

We do not claim that everyone's senility will be prevented or reversed. Not every apparent senile is actually senile as several conditions will produce a similar clinical syndrome. Each condition will require specific treatment, and some are irreversible and will not respond. Our therapeutic program will harm no one but will help many, especially if started early. Other pathological conditions must be ruled out, of course, lest total reliance on our program discourages specific treatment from being used.

We anticipate this volume will not only light a fire under geriatricians, medical scientists and nutritionists, but will be followed by a massive research effort to test the whole program on a large scale. Such research won't be done to convince *us* but to prove the program's value to skeptical physicians who find large studies with statistical tables more impressive.

Meanwhile, since life is short and untreated senility is unrelenting in its march, we suggest you not wait for the decades required to persuade our medical schools and medical societies. It is your sanity which is at stake while the physician waits for hard clinical evidence.

A. HOFFER, M.D., Ph.D.

1

AGING IS INEVITABLE
BUT NOT SENILITY

> *Growing old is just a process of getting tired. Soon I shall doze off, and then fall asleep. How beautiful to stretch oneself out!*
>> —Malcolm Muggeridge, *The New York Times*, April 24, 1978

Senility Reversal of the Senior Mrs. Hoffer

IN 1954, my wife Rose and I had completed our plans for a three-month tour of psychiatric research centers of Europe. The trip came about after the Rockefeller Foundation had awarded my research group a large financial grant. Over a three-year period, we were responsible for investigating the bio-chemical basis for schizophrenia. It was an awesome responsibility, and I was eager to begin its development.

Accompanying the Foundation's grant, however, was an offer made which I could not refuse. The philanthropists asked me to tour research centers throughout Europe as their guest and take on the role of "Rockefeller Traveling Fellow." It was necessary for me to make the trip before beginning the new expanded research program because any information gleaned abroad might be useful in my group's investigations.

As it turned out, this trip played both a direct and indirect role in the formation of a highly successful antisenility nutrition program. A family circumstance

7

provided me with the dramatic instance of senility reversal using orthomolecular methods. The first patient for whom I prescribed orthomolecular nutrition for the treatment and reversal of the senile syndrome was my own mother, Mrs. Clara Hoffer.

My mother was then sixty-six years old and laboring under severe emotional stress. My father, a year older, had retired from his farm to a house in Regina, the largest city and capital of Saskatchewan, Canada. However, he stopped work only for the winters. My dad had never been happy in a city, which he found boring and distasteful. He preferred his own domain—the country—where he never felt bored.

Stress was present for both mother and dad because he was the victim of inoperable cancer of the prostate, and was dying.

Mother preferred to be in the city. She felt lonely and insecure on the farm, especially during the dark winter. Winters in Saskatchewan farm country are harsh, cold, long and lonely.

The conflict in emotions, consequently, created enormous stress for her. It was not only that she knew dad had but a few months left—she dreaded the loneliness, miserableness, and boredom of residing in the country.

I did what I could to help them remain in the city by trying to give dad a sense of purpose. For a while, I kept my father busy doing a little laboratory work by having him grow oat plants. The idea was to germinate these plants in urine from schizophrenic patients and after a few days to measure the length of all the rootlets and stems. One of the plant hormones, an indole, changed the ratio of roots to stem. I hoped that the toxin we were certain was present in schizophrenic urine and which we thought was an indole, would alter the ratio in the same way as the plant hormone, the auxins. Thus, I set my father onto the project as my investigator.

During my last visit with my parents before sailing for

Europe, Mother complained to me about how sick she was. Without question, she was having physical and mental problems: losing vision in one eye, a failing memory, swollen and painful joints, and the feeling of pain when moving from place to place. Also, she had lost interest in what was going on; forgot names, addresses, and phone numbers; repeated things she already had said; forgot recent events; had vivid remembrance of her early life; and showed a rigidity in her pattern of living. In short, mother was showing signs of senility. The question in my mind was could I, as a psychiatrist, provide her with any relief?

I had no doubt that she was developing the beginning changes characteristic of the senile syndrome that hit so many older people. I "knew" there was no treatment for it, much as most traditional physicians today "know" that the condition is not reversible. In good conscience, I felt the need to offer my mother some kind of help, even if it was merely a placebo. A placebo, you may know, is an indifferent substance, in the form of a medicine, given for its suggestive effect.

Previously, I had already completed two double blind controlled comparison experiments using placebos with Dr. Humphry Osmond, the first such experiments ever accomplished in psychiatry. Indeed, I was quite familiar with the placebo effect, which in England was then called the "dummy" effect. Its success was ascribed to the faith and hope of the patient in a remedy for the alleviation of his symptoms. The science of placebology, in 1954, had just briefly flashed across the scene and was beginning to develop.

A placebo was believed to be more effective if the supposed good effect could be dramatized. This was achieved by a persuasive and charismatic healer, by the proper use of suggestive factors or by some remarkable property of the "drug" being given. It occurred to me that the B-vitamin nicotinic acid (also known as *niacin*) would be the ideal placebo. It had all the desired properties.

Nicotinic acid was a familiar friend to me. I had been using it for two years with patients and taken it myself to study its effect. My research staff, who were enthusiastic about our studies, also were trying it out on themselves. It was completely safe, but I found it did cause a pronounced facial flush which eventually dissipated. Although I did not know it at the time, nicotinic acid lowers blood cholesterol and triglycerides, which is advantageous for the anti-atherosclerotic effect. Several years before, this B vitamin was also discovered to be curative for the more common forms of arthritis by William Kaufman, M.D.[1,2]

I had no reason to suspect that nicotinic acid would be of any value in preventing, treating, or reversing senility. While I did establish that it was exceedingly useful for treating schizophrenics who were not fixed into typical chronic cases, my chief reason for giving it to my mother was strictly for its placebo effect. I thought she would acquire faith and find hope from experiencing the niacin flush.

I gave her a supply for three months with the advice to take one gram after each meal. The possible side effects were carefully outlined, and my mother was prepared for them.

About six weeks later, my wife and I received a very cheerful and enthusiastic letter in London from the Senior Mrs. Hoffer. She wrote that she was feeling much better—so much so that she had regained her vision. Her neuralgia, another complaint which chronically disabled her, was gone entirely. She said her memory was normal. Her arthritic pains were gone completely, and the four small arthritic bumps on her knuckles called "Heberden's nodes" were disappearing.

I was pleased with my mother's report but frankly felt credulous, and expressed this feeling to Rose. I could not believe it was any kind of real recovery. My assumption was that the powerful placebo effect had clouded the woman's own assessment of her health. Furthermore, my prior medical indoctrination was that Heberden's nodes never went away.

When we arrived home in July 1954, Rose and I drove to my parents' farm near Hoffer, Saskatchewan, where I had been born and raised. Immediately upon seeing my mother, I realized her mental and physical responses were no placebo effect. Mother was cheerful, relaxed, at ease, mentally alert, quickly responsive with accurate answers to any questions I asked, and she moved with the step of a young woman. The arthritis which had begun to cripple her hands and hips had disappeared. There is no denying that an arthritic condition which had begun to pull her fingers out—the typical ulnar deviation—was no longer present. Her hands were supple, flexible, and free of pain. The little Heberden's bumps had gone away altogether. Her joints were much softer, flatter, and the bony prominences on her fingers were receding back to skin level.

I thought long and hard about my mother's mental and physical improvement. It caused me to suspect that what I "knew" to be the irreversibility of senility and the physical changes in which it was developed were not true at all. If just one person responded to the ingestion of nicotinic acid, then others would also respond. For although we are all unique bio-chemical individuals, we are not *that* unique. The only problem was to find out how many others would also respond to niacin, and how the doctor and patient could decide this in advance. I investigated over time and followed through with careful studies. My suspicions have now been confirmed: Niacin supplementation is a definite antisenility therapy. My conclusion is that this remarkable vitamin should be incorporated as a significant component of any treatment program against senility.

My mother was in good mental health until she sustained a stroke five years ago, dying one month later at the age of eighty-seven. During this interval of twenty-one years, she continued to take regular doses of nicotinic acid, ranging from 1 to 4 grams per day. I had added vitamin C and vitamin E as well as other nutrients (described in Chapter Seven) to her antisenility dietary program. She maintained an active life for the whole of this time. She participated in all family social activities and wrote her memoirs. In fact, in collaboration with her daughter, Fannie Kahan, my mother published two books, one dealing with her early farm experiences in Canada, and the other dealing with my father's agricultural experiences in Europe and in Saskatchewan where he had arrived in 1905 to start farming on a homestead.

There is no doubt in my mind that nicotinic acid saved Mother from senility, physical weakness, insecurity, and the terrors of living in a nursing home. I testify that certain nutrients combined with this niacin permitted her to age without senility.

There are other cases as well. We shall describe them in the chapters that follow, since among them, you may find a model of senility reversal which you might be able to match to your own family situation.

Aging Is Inevitable but Not Senility

It isn't difficult to distinguish an old person from a young person. Throughout life, a variety of changes occur in our bodies which appear to be inevitable. These aging changes reflect biochemical reactions in the cells and anatomical alterations in the organs. The many changes don't happen at the same rate in all the organs, and they take place at varying times from one person to the next. Rather striking, in fact, is the remarkable variation in aging among individuals and the organs in the same individual. Some are aged by the time they are forty years old; others appear youthful at eighty. Some organs—a kidney or the stomach of a person—could probably go on functioning normally for another few decades, but the heart gives out and causes early death.

Aging is inevitable and is inevitably followed by death. The rate at which aging occurs, however, is not highly correlated with age itself as measured in years. It is this flexible relationship—inevitable aging at variable rates of time—which makes this book possible and necessary.

If everyone inevitably aged and deteriorated at the same rate, it would mean that all of us had been programmed in the same way. We might age, deteriorate, and die much like the self-destruct devices so loved by some science fiction novelists. There would be no reason to think that anything could be done to change one's life pattern. But we *can* change our lives and be the masters of our destiny. We have the ability to approach the full span of human existence—120 years—with alert, creative, memory-filled minds.

Around us we see many people die old, but not senile. Such observations are encouraging, even inspiring. They support our belief that it is possible to prepare a nutritional environment which permits nearly everyone who so wishes to reach the same desirable state, that is, to age without senility. A good deal of evidence exists showing such a nutritional environment is feasible right now, and not in the golden future suggested by medical research scientists.

Our claim is that no one needs to depend just on the variability of the aging process. The information that we supply in this book will permit every reader to take steps to decrease his or her rate of aging. Put to use, our nutritional program will allow the reversal of some of the changes having taken place already.

While this nutritional information won't necessarily make anyone live longer, it will increase the potential for a healthier life expectancy. It will improve the quality of life in the more advanced age bracket. Why? How? To illustrate: a youthful individual at seventy is more apt to avoid accidents such as being run down by a car than an aged and deteriorated person of seventy. This will be, even for no other reason than the more active seventy-year-old's ability to dodge out of the path of an oncoming automobile. And, he'll have the presence of mind to do so. A non-senile seventy-year-old person will be enjoying a fullness in living that is sorely lacking for someone of the same age suffering from senile dementia.

To repeat, the program of nutrients we will recommend here can improve the quality of life when you incorporate those nutrients into your daily diet. Even though the aim would be laudable, we aren't deluded by the longing to prolong life. We mean only to show the non-inevitability of senility. Our recommendations, if followed, will ensure that at death, no matter the reason or age at which it occurs, there will be no, or very few, indications of senility.

It has been said that "old age can become an expression of human experience. It can be rich, varied, colorful, and in turn enriching; or it can be impoverished, empty, and only serve to emphasize the futility of life." For the elderly of today, reality is best described by the latter possibility. With this book, our aim is to transpose it into the former— a journey toward love without any fixed point. As the poet Keats put it:

> And like a newborn spirit did he pass
> Through the green evening quiet in the sun.

The Incidence of Old Age and Senility

The import of our message knows no bounds, for the incidence of old age and its associated senility is steadily on the rise. Today we may be living slightly longer, but we are not enjoying healthier lives.

Anyone reaching age forty-five today has no better chance of attaining age ninety than had he lived one hundred years ago. The major improvements for longevity have taken place in younger people. Older people who live longer do so not because they are healthier, but because medicine is more skillful at keeping them alive. There is no corresponding improvement in the health of the elderly. In fact, up to now, aging and senility have been developing at an accelerating pace.

This last statement is proven by Kraus, Spasoff, Beattie, Holden, Lawson, Rodenburg and Woodcock (1977).[3] They showed that in the United States 1.2 percent of the age group sixty-five to seventy-four, 5.2 percent of the age group seventy-five to eighty-four, and 20.3 percent of the eighty-five and over age group were in special nursing homes equipped for treating senility. Of the last group, 31 percent were bedfast, 11 percent were chairfast, 74 percent had three or more chronic illnesses, and 71 percent were senile.

Between 1961 and 1971, Canada's population increased by 18 percent. But the population increase in the sixty-five to seventy-four years group was 21 percent; in the seventy-five to eighty-four years group it was 26 percent; in the eighty-five and over years group it was 70 percent.

In 1972, 137,000 Canadians lived to be eighty-five or older, while ten times this number attained this age in the United States. But 70 percent of these elderly Americans were senile. In 1975, geriatrics occupied one-third of all hospital beds for the acutely ill in the United States at a cost of $118.7 billion, and during that year, 1.2 million elderly were in nursing homes. One fourth of the drugs taken were consumed by older Americans.

The Office of Human Development of the U.S. Department of Health, Education and Welfare projects 71 million old people by the year 2035. One-third will be over seventy-five, one-tenth will be over eighty-five. By the year 2000, the aged will constitute 20 percent of the national population. Right now, one of every nine Americans is a senior citizen who typically can expect to live another sixteen years, according to the Senate Committee on Aging. Social Security records reveal that 10,690 Americans are at least one hundred years old. About 75 percent of all Americans now reach the age of sixty-five. Florida leads the states in percentage of population sixty-five or older with 14 percent. Alaska, Hawaii, and Utah are at the bottom with 7.9 percent.

Three percent of the population over age sixty-five have psychiatric problems leading to limitation of their activities. The senile are included in this figure. If the same rate continues, we will have two million people suffering from senility in the next ten years. Yet, this statistic is an underestimate since the increase appears to be geometric, not arithmetic.

Kraus, Spasoff, and their associates compared two groups of people aged eighty-five or older. One group consisted of those applying for admission to special nursing homes and the other group consisted of those living independently in the community. Certain physical changes forced the first group to apply for admission. Pathological malfunctioning of body systems made it impossible for old people to live alone, or created intolerable circumstances for others.

One-third of the elderly applicants suffered serious vision and hearing impediments compared to one-fourth of the independents. One-fifth of the applicants had trouble controlling urinary or excretory functions while less than one-tenth of the independents experienced these problems. Of the applicants, 67 percent needed help in bathing, 44 percent with dressing, and 25 percent in going to the toilet. None of the independents required any of this kind of help. Of the applicants, one-third were disoriented with respect to space and time; none of the independents experienced this disorientation. If a similar study were made on those eighty-five and older already in institutions, there would undoubtedly be even more pathology.

Clearly, if we could prevent deterioration in seeing and hearing, maintain bowel and bladder control, prevent disorientation, and do away with physical infirmity, society would have almost no applicants for admission to special nursing homes.

We are convinced that a major decrease in senility can be effected even though there will be some in whom this program will not work. Still, we can start. In time, we will approach a state where senility is considered a failure by society in providing a healthy personal lifestyle and proper medical care.

What Is Senility?

Senility is in no way the same as aging. Everybody ages, but only some people become senile. Senility is the term applied to destructive changes in the functioning cells of the brain. It is a brain disease and a mental disease. While there are senile physical changes as well, they are not always present in the brain of the senile person.

In the brain of a young healthy adult, there are about 12 billion neurons, the cells that send nerve impulses through the body. As part of the aging process each day, the brain loses about 100,000 neurons. They get used up and die; most probably this results from the intake of toxic substances. After sixty or more years of losing these irreplaceable brain cells, an uneven pattern develops in the individual's thinking. His mind wanders and he may no longer be able to retain near-term memories. In a word, he becomes senile.

Geriatric specialists estimate that 15 percent of people sixty-five to seventy-five years old and 25 percent of those seventy-five and older are senile. As we mentioned before, the number is growing. Scientists generally don't recognize any particular reason for the greater incidence of senility. Our claim is that it derives from a certain malnutrition.

The word *senility* is derived from the Latin meaning *old*. It is a condition characterized by memory loss, particularly for recent events, loss of ability to do simple problems in addition and subtraction, possible incipient blindness, and confusion as to where the person is, how he got there, when he arrived, and why he is there at all. There is no specific laboratory test that helps someone diagnose the presence of senility. It is strictly an impressionistic decision made by an objective third party—often a physician.

Some of the newest medical instrumentation such as a computerized axial tomogram (CAT scanner) shows a shrunken brain on X ray, and this has helped to make a diagnosis of senility. The CAT scan alone, however, is not yet considered a verified diagnostic test for this condition.

It's important to make an accurate diagnosis for senility because many different health problems can produce symptoms that mimic senility. Some elderly people are falsely labeled senile when their symptoms come from depression, a malfunctioning thyroid gland, pernicious anemia, the effects of drugs such as bromides, or from a variety of other conditions, which may be treatable. We will discuss these differential diagnoses in depth in the next chapter.

It has been thought for years that hardening of the arteries in the brain was the cause of senility. During the last eight years, research studies have turned up that sclerosis of the brain's blood vessels plays less of a role in the condition than had been thought previously. On the basis of arteriosclerosis, senility tends to produce worsening symptoms episodically. Geriatricians have now changed their thinking and believe the bulk of cases come from senile dementia, a disease more common in women. *Senile dementia* is characterized by the gradual, unrelenting deterioration of the mind. Geriatricians assume the cause is unknown and the pathology irreversible. We say that neither of these assumptions is correct.

When senility develops in a forty- or fifty-year-old person, it is then called *presenile dementia*. Doctors pin a pathological label on the patient in such an age group and call the condition *Alzheimer's disease* or *Pick's disease*. In Alzheimer's disease, the shrinkage occurs throughout the brain.

In Pick's disease, the changes are more localized. Pathologists have claimed that since Alzheimer's disease is indistinguishable on autopsy from the shrunken, senile brain, Alzheimer's might be merely the early onset of the more common form of senility.

At the beginning of research into the gross and microscopic anatomy of the brain, medical scientists believed that senile brains underwent characteristic alterations which could be identified. The pathologists looked for them: softness of brain tissue, obliteration of cells, lines of demarcation between viable matter and mush. In some cases, brains from senile folk were in fact quite deteriorated, but to a more surprising degree, most senile brains were normal. There were even plenty of nonseniles who had mushy-looking brains. The relationship between the amount of pathology in the brain and the presence of senility turned out inconclusive. The theories of the beginning medical scientists were dashed into nothingness.

If a large chunk of an individual's brain was destroyed by a tumor, a stroke or a head wound, we could obviously be justified in expecting a major defect in the person's performance. However, these kinds of changes are quite different from those present in a senile person. The senile patient has distinguishing signs of memory loss, an inability to store new information, and certain personality quirks.

There being a dissimilarity between the brain-damaged person and a senile person, is there any damage whatever in the senile brain? We believe there is—biochemical damage rather than mechanical damage. The basis of our nutritional program to prevent senility is that senile defects manifest themselves from biochemical alterations which have not yet been entirely identified. Only a small portion of the pathology is known. Some correlation prevails between the degree of biochemical pathology and the degree of senility.

Biochemical Changes Differ from Physical Changes

It is reasonable that senile changes in the brain should be different from physical senile changes seen in other organs. Some body organs are subject to mechanical tearing. They suffer from wear!

For instance, bones bear a great deal of weight and pull away from muscles. The heart is in constant motion. Other organs such as liver, kidney, pancreas, and brain are subject to minor mechanical strain. But, the only mechanical strain in the brain arises from the unmomentous pulsation of its blood vessels.

Since it is passive, the brain ought to be one of the last organs in the body to deteriorate. Only ions and molecules are transmitted to and fro across its membranes. Such particles do not wear down tissue. Logically, as long as the molecular state of the brain remains intact, its function will remain intact.

The biochemical activity of the brain differs entirely from the physical functionings of the other body organs.

Every organ has a special function. The liver is a chemical factory for changing molecules. The lung places blood in close contact with air so it can eliminate carbon dioxide and take up oxygen. The kidney purifies blood; the bladder stores urine.

The brain has its unique function as well. It must coordinate all the various components of the body in order for the body to function as a whole and not as a committee of individual parts. The brain must also relate to our two main human environments, the psychosocial and the biophysical. To carry out this very elaborate, intricate function, the brain must be in direct contact with every section of the body, must interpret and react to all the signals speeding to it, and initiate appropriate stimuli to regulate and control the body.

Most of us are unaware of the brain's activity and luckily so. If we had to pay attention to even a tiny fraction of its activity, we would not be able to function. Some people are disabled simply from being constantly aware of their heart beat. Feeling heart palpitations can be disconcerting. The basic automatic activity of the brain provides us with stability, which is absolutely essential if we are to live within our psychosocial and biophysical environments.

The second main activity of this remarkable organ concerns our senses. We are aware of seeing, hearing, tasting, touching, smelling, and our body cognizance. We know, for instance, how the body is oriented with respect to gravity. Awareness of our external world is mediated through our senses. This is called *perception*. It is more than having images accurately focused upon the retina, or of recording sound in our ears. Such signals must be transmitted to the brain and be recognized. Perception is quite a complex phenomenon.

The Demands of Perception

Perception demands recognition and reaction; it also requires thinking. And, one demand tends to impinge on another. Each percept is identified as either something trivial to be ignored, or as something that requires concentrated attention. It is a decision the brain usually makes instantaneously, depending upon the person's experience with similar percepts in the past.

Perception also is dependent on one's alertness. Many hyperactive children are too alert, too distractable, and apparently are unable to decide what is trivial or not trivial. A slight rustle here, an object there, demands their full attention even if only for a few seconds. Such reactions to distractions may be totally inappropriate. On the other hand, a hyperactive's attention may be so diminished that even an important event such as a car bearing down on the child is ignored. Diminished attention may terminate the child's life.

Important, or interesting objects or circumstances require reaction. The reaction may vary from giving continuing attention to the phenomenon, to fleeing from it in fear in another direction. Again, rapid decisions are needed which will be based on the past as well as on genetic behavior patterns.

Failure of the Brain to Function

When the brain fails to function, its failure may affect all four areas of living—perception, thinking, feeling, and behavior. Usually one area will be more affected than others. From such functional changes we derive syndromes. A *syndrome* is an aggregate of signs and symptoms associated with any morbid process, which constitute together the picture of a disease. The syndrome determines which treatment is most appropriate.

A combination of changes in perception and in thinking including visions, voices and inappropriate responses constitute the schizophrenic syndrome.

When disturbances in memory, disorientation for person, time and place, and confusion are also present, we have the syndrome of delirium.

When the main changes are in mood, we are dealing with the neuroses—anxiety, depression and tensions.

Senility is a very peculiar syndrome consisting of changes in memory, disorientation and confusion. If changes in perception were present in senility, it would be a delirium; there are no perceptual changes.

A cardsorting, 145-item questionnaire which identifies and adds up an individual's sensory and time distortions, the Hoffer-Osmond Diagnostic (HOD) test, has been administered to a large number of senile patients.[4,5] Their perceptual scores are almost invariably low, and they deny the presence of illusions and hallucinations. This has happened so frequently, one's conclusion must be that the senile patient does not have perceptual disturbances and paranoid thoughts. When illusions and hallucinations are present, the examiner should consider that either schizophrenia or delirium is present, but this is not the apparent case in senility.

Memory Loss in the Senile Patient

The thinking changes in senility are of a peculiar sort. The main problem is in the area of memory. Furthermore, there is recent evidence which suggests that perhaps it is the ability to learn which is altered. Memory for recent events is mainly modified. You might experience the strange phenomenon that the senile patient may not remember what he had for breakfast, or whether he even had breakfast at all. Nevertheless, he can describe a memorable meal he had eaten many years before.

The ability to impress an event so that it can later be recalled seems to be damaged in the senile person. The evidence which points to a learning defect rather than a simple memory defect was first pointed out to us by Professor Edwin Boyle, Jr., M.D., when he was research director of the Miami Heart Institute. At that time, he was investigating the effect of hyperbaric oxygen on those patients who were becoming senile or already had been senile for several years.

Dr. Boyle gave his patients thirty-minute treatments by placing them in a chamber containing two atmospheres pressure of pure oxygen. A large number of senile people were studied in this way, each receiving the oxygen treatment. They underwent five hyperbaric sessions each week for two weeks, but not on weekends. In some cases, senility appeared to have been vanquished, for patients formerly hopelessly senile became suddenly normal. They were able to remember not only the past but experiences which had occurred in the present, as well. Unfortunately, their senility began to recur in several weeks. Each person returned to his pretreatment senile level by the end of a few months. The benefit was only temporary.

The result of this bit of experimentation is of vital importance. It does not suggest that hyperbaric therapy is useless, but that it alone is not the answer to senility. Hyperbaric oxygen will provide a useful therapeutic effect when a way is discovered to maintain the patient's overall state of health. Also, the experiment proves that what the senile person learned could still be remembered. It is new learning that had disappeared. This further points to the possible biochemical error which creates senility.

We agree with Professor Boyle when he declares that senility is basically a loss of learning ability. Still, in this book, we shall discuss memory loss as the chief happenstance of the condition.

At the beginning, it is not too difficult for a person whose brain is deteriorating to compensate for memory losses. The early senile may write important things down or ask others to jog his memory. Memory loss remains a minor inconvenience. Since intellect remains unimpaired, one can compensate also by making excuses (except the statement "I forgot" is not acceptable). The individual can also fabricate—make up events or stories to satisfy the person to whom the senile is talking. This sort of story telling is often done skillfully. For this reason, it is essential to have a relative present who knows the truth. A spouse can readily correct the patient's confabulated or minimized information.

It is usual for preseniles to admit a few memory problems, but to minimize them. A memory problem may wax and wane until it finally becomes irreversibly fixed. It is mandatory for treatment to be started before it is fixed; the longer therapy is delayed, the less significant are the results.

Memory loss is not too difficult for the presenile if there is no disorientation. However, if an individual becomes lost in time, confused geographically, or fails to recognize himself or others, memory loss becomes impossible to deal with. This will give rise to the trying circumstances of witnessing the senile person wandering away from home, getting lost even in familiar surroundings, or getting hurt on the street. It is a sad occurrence, especially for someone who formerly "had it all together."

Senile people equally lose themselves in time. The past becomes their life; the present is an irritant; there is no future. They fail to recognize their spouses, sons and daughters. They relive what happened to them many years before. They are quite helpless psychologically and require shelter, protection and devoted nursing care.

Although society accepts its inevitability, we no longer believe senility is as inescapable as death. Our change of mind is based upon what we have seen in the practice of orthomolecular psychiatry. This is direct observable evidence, the only kind admissible in a court of law. It is not hearsay evidence, which is not admissible. Science and medicine have a different attitude toward these two modes of facts or evidence. Too often, admissible evidence, that which has been witnessed personally, is disregarded as subjective, while hearsay evidence, that which has been heard from others, is admissible. Perhaps, this is why medicine is so frequently embroiled in useless debates. The field of orthomolecular psychiatry has suffered from this peculiar regard for forms of evidence. Traditional psychiatry has turned a deaf ear to orthomolecular practices and the senile have suffered from this disregard.

The proponents of orthomolecular psychiatry depend upon hearsay, too, but rely much more upon personal, direct observations. In most cases, hearsay evidence serves merely to arouse interest. The conclusion that orthomolecular therapy is effective against senility is based entirely on direct personal observations—upon the only evidence admissible by any court. We will present our evidence in the following chapters. You can judge whether or not senility is reversible. Categorically, we say that senility does not have to be the inevitable result of aging.

Bergson, the famous philosopher, has compared the aging process with a sand-clock: in the upper part are the good substances and in the lower part, the bad ones. While the first diminishes, the second increases.

We cannot reverse the sand-clock, but thanks to several discoveries about nutrient dependencies, we are able to reduce the outflow of the sand, to increase its upper part and diminish the lower.

References for Chapter One

1. Kaufman, W. *Common Form of Niacinamide Deficiency Disease: Aniacinamidosis.* New Haven, Conn.: Yale University Press, 1943.

2. Kaufman, W. *The Common Form of Joint Dysfunction: Its Incidence and Treatment.* Brattleboro, Vermont: E. L. Hildreth and Co., 1949.

3. Kraus, A.S.; Spasoff, R.A.; Beattie, E.J.; Holden, D.E.W.; Lawson, J.S.; Rodenburg, M.; and Woodcock, G.M. The health of the very aged. *Canadian Medical Association Journal* 116:1007-1009, 1977.

4. Hoffer, A.; Kelm, H.; and Osmond, H. *The Hoffer-Osmond Diagnostic Test.* Huntington, New York: Robert E. Krieger Publishing Co., 1975.
    Test kit available from Behavior Science Press,
    P.O. Box A, G., University, Alabama 35486

5. Hoffer, A. and Osmond, H. A card sorting test helpful in making psychiatric diagnosis. *Journal of Neuropsychiatry* 2: 306-330, 1961.

2

NORMAL AGING, PREMATURE AGING AND PSEUDOSENILITY

You can't retire from life and you shouldn't. You should use the four great chords of mental health: the ability to love, the ability to work, the ability to play, and the ability to think critically. And if you can achieve this, all with a sense of humor or playfulness, then you're likely to lead a very much more satisfactory life than you otherwise would.

—Ashley Montague, *Psychology Today*, August 1977

The Biology of Normal Aging

DURING THE FIRST WEEK of May, 1977, a special tribunal of seven appellate court justices ordered the retirement of California Supreme Court Justice Marshall F. McComb. He was declared senile. The tribunal was following the recommendation of the California Commission on Judicial Performance, which had heard evidence of the justice's inability to perform his duties. Charges were first filed against Justice McComb in April, 1976.

This Supreme Court Justice's colleagues found that he sometimes fell asleep on the bench, read magazines in court, or did physical exercises while counting aloud and walked out of judicial conferences that he described as "talk, talk, talk; squawk, squawk, squawk; yak, yak, yak." Justice McComb had fifty years of judicial service behind him, and the tribunal ruled that it was time for him to retire.

His wife was named conservator for her husband after she testified that he could no longer care for himself or his property.[1]

Justice McComb is an example of the gradual onset of senility accenting the peculiarities that have existed in a personality for years but were repressed during earlier years. He had a disease of the brain, but it was not caused by his growing old. It's just that the diseases commonly associated with old age are simply those which require decades to develop and usually don't show up in young people. Our society's misconception is that when you're young and get sick, it's labeled "illness," but when you're old and get sick, it's called "aging." Sickness and aging, however, are two different states of being.

As we grow older, the 60 trillion cells in our bodies gradually change. Each cell has a limited life—after which it reproduces itself through a process called "mitosis" or doubling. Then the cell dies. Thus, at any given second, thousands of your cells may be dying, yet thousands are also being reborn, some faster than others. For example, while fat cells may reproduce slowly, skin cells reproduce approximately every ten hours. As mentioned in the last chapter, the notable exception to this constant cell replacement is found in the brain. The moment any of us are born, we have our lifetime maximum number of brain cells, and when these become worn out, they are never replaced. By age 35, each person loses 100,000 brain cells a day, but because the initial surplus is so great, the loss is scarcely noticeable.

As you grow older, you may discover some changes taking place in your senses, energy level, and the functioning of different parts of the body. For instance, your sense of taste and smell will diminish. By age sixty, most people have lost 50 percent of their taste buds, especially if they smoke cigarettes; the ability to smell reduces by 40 percent. You may find that your muscles lack tone, especially facial muscles and those in the back of the arms. Hair and nails start to break more easily and may lack luster. Skin becomes dry and loses its elasticity, taking on a wrinkled appearance. Blood pressure rises, arteries plug and breathing takes more effort. There are, in fact, a vast number of characteristics which constitute aging. We shall describe them in detail in the next section. Before doing that, however, let us add a note of encouragement.

- There does exist within ourselves an indefinable "clock of aging."
- There is an excellent chance of discovering the location of this clock, and intervening in its mechanisms to our advantage.
- This can happen within a few decades if the proper emphasis on research is advanced.

Characteristics Which Constitute Aging

As we stated, in aging, gross changes take place that are characteristic of physiological wear and tear. The physical appearance of aging is all too familiar, but the subjective interpretation of how old someone is apparently does vary with the age of the viewer, too. Interestingly, as we age ourselves, the people we recognize in the sixty to seventy year population don't seem quite as old as we formerly found them to appear when we were a few decades younger ourselves.

The characteristic changes of aging include all the organs and tissues of the body.

Skin Changes: The skin loses its elasticity; a lifted skin fold settles back slowly rather than immediately regaining its normal position as once it had done. Elderly skin is dry, wrinkled, and may take on a parchment quality. Localized pigmented plaques develop. The skin gets fragile and bruises easily. These are changes not likely to arise solely from aging, but from many years of malnutrition, insult from the sun, and other factors. Such skin is able to be restored to its original elasticity and health from receiving proper nutritional treatment.

Derived from skin and having similar nutritional requirements, hair will take on specific aging characteristics of its own. The greying of hair takes place either early or late in life, depending on one's genes and blood flow to the scalp. Perspiration glands and oil glands on the head work less efficiently with age, and hair becomes thin even when no actual baldness exists. The nails take on a brittleness and ridges as well as discoloration occur.

Since the skin layer is the largest organ of the body, any observer can guess correctly that these outward changes of hair and skin indicate equally major changes in the rest of the body.

Muscle Changes: Muscles lose many fibers, and the fibers remaining in an aged person become weaker in strength. Arms and legs tend to reduce muscle mass and look thinner. Less muscle mass may also come from the individual's associated lessening of activity.

In the heart muscle, there is an increase in the yellow-brown pigment, lipofuscin, which is one of the lipochromes. The total ribonucleic acid (RNA) usually present in cells varies inversely with the amount of lipochrome. As lipochrome continues to deposit with age, RNA decreases steadily. Even though little is known as to how to reverse these aging changes in the heart, it has been suggested by the two Canadian heart specialists, Drs. Wilfrid Shute and Evan Shute, that vitamin E may be helpful in the diminution of lipochrome deposits. Furthermore, extra lipochrome is laid down in the neurones of laboratory rats that are deficient in vitamin E. Another report says that magnesium orotate and kavain, a food supplement prepared from kava kava, both prevent the deposition of lipochrome.

Skeletal Changes: The skeletons of elderly people shrink with age. Deformations due to osteoporosis develop when calcium leaches from bones leaving them thinner, weaker and more fragile. Approximately 25 percent of women and 6 percent of men over age sixty-five suffer from this calcium deficiency. It is believed to be derived from a lack of vitamin D-3 and sunlight, along with a calcium deficiency. Geriatrics who seldom leave their rooms are most apt to suffer from osteoporosis, but inadequate exercise is also a major factor.

The skeleton continues to remodel itself in its adaptation to stress. New bone is laid down to reinforce stressed areas and unstressed bone gets resorbed. On the one hand, bones used continually become much stronger but conversely, infrequently stressed bones lose substance. With the prevalence of osteoporosis, the elderly suffer fractures of the head of the femur, hips, and the vertebral body even from trivial trauma. Obviously, the best preventative of osteoporosis is a sufficient intake of calcium, vitamin D-3, and the daily use of one's skeleton.

Astronauts in a weightless environment, as with the elderly who don't exercise, suffer from some osteoporosis. This condition tends to repair itself as soon as normal skeletal stress becomes possible again. The astronauts' experience indicates that calcium can be removed from the bones so quickly that it will settle down with associated phosphorus in soft tissues such as the kidney.

Cardiovascular Changes: Aging of the vascular system shows up as an increase in atherosclerotic plaques in the blood vessels. The walls of arteries grow inelastic; heart valves become thicker; and an increase in fat and connective tissue gather around the heart.

Because of an excess intake of sugar and salt among the elderly (whose taste buds seem to require more flavoring from a diminished taste for food), blood pressure tends to increase. For seventy- to seventy-nine-year-old men, the absolute upper limit of normal blood pressure is 205/104, systolic over diastolic. For women in the same age range, it is 215/106. Men between the ages of eighty to eighty-nine have a systolic/diastolic upper limit normal blood pressure of 215/108, and women have 230/110, according to Sir Ferguson Anderson, Professor of Geriatric Medicine, Glasgow School of Medicine, and the 1977 president of the British Medical Association.

We urge that lower limits be used as a basis for recording normal blood pressures in the elderly, not as an indication for antihypertensive drug treatment, but as a means for reassessment of the patient's nutrition and activity status. There is no strong relationship between blood pressure and mortality until the blood pressure exceeds 200/120. High blood pressure is a major risk factor for stroke.

Kidney Changes: The reserve capacity of the kidneys tends to decrease to 50 percent of what was once present, but usually there is enough to maintain correct fluid and mineral balance. This is made more difficult for many older people because they drink too little water. About three decades ago, a brief survey of newly admitted senile patients to a mental hospital in Saskatchewan revealed that 25 percent were there as a result of dehydration. These patients possessed too low an awareness of thirst. They only needed an increased fluid intake to get well physically.

The elderly person should make an effort to drink enough water even if he or she isn't thirsty. Perhaps a zinc deficiency, which is the cause of a decreased taste for food, is also responsible for the diminished sense of thirst.

Lung Changes: The lungs' self-cleaning function reduces with age. Consequently, an older person's capacity to exchange respiratory gases such as oxygen substituted for carbon dioxide in the blood is decreased. When the muscles get weaker, the chest wall becomes less elastic and inspiration is not as deep.

Changes in the Central Nervous System: By age ninety, symmetrical cerebral atrophy sets in with the brain losing about one-quarter of its weight. The fissures (sulci) on the surface of the brain widen and the brain ventricles slowly enlarge. If there is a sudden enlargement, or more enlargement than would be expected by the regular aging process, it is possible that a blockage of the cerebrospinal fluid, a hydrocephalus, is present. Such a hydrocephalus can be a cause of senility and should be treated surgically by introducing a bypass around the source of brain pressure.

Up to 30 percent of the neurones in a geriatric brain may be lost. The extracellular space in the brain vault decreases and senile plaques form. Alzheimer's disease, a form of early senility, is associated with neurofibrillary changes. They occur first in the hippocampus, which is the complex, internally convoluted structure of the cortical mantle of the cerebral hemisphere. Much later, the changes take place in the neocortex. Giving laboratory animals aluminum salts has reproduced these same kinds of changes.

When neurones are examined microscopically using Golgi impregnation techniques, they are observed to have lost their normal shape. They become lumpy and gradually have fewer dendrites. Neuromelanins, the dark brown pigments derived from noradrenalin and adrenalin, increase in quantity.

With these changes, we would expect malfunctioning of the brain, and this does occur even though the brain has reserve capacity and can compensate for a long time.

Until 1900, it was assumed there was a good correlation between senility and organic brain changes. Between 1930 and 1950, scientists questioned these assumptions. Since then it has become apparent that there is a threshold effect. Morphological changes occur slowly but impairment of function manifests itself when a critical level of pathology is reached. Senility is a designation of that pathology.

The Psycho-Physiology of Premature Aging

Before senility actually sets in, many people in Western industrialized countries undergo premature aging. It is an illness which is, for the most part, neglected by European and North American medicine. This sickness does not kill in the obvious way. It cannot be described in a clear manner, and no postmortem indicates its presence. Rather, premature aging is a psycho-physiological disease of our modern civilization manifested by a number of subjective symptoms which are constantly present and commonly accepted. They are influenced by heredity, ecological conditions, the way of living, and past diseases.

When examining a man of fifty, his doctor may find his heart to be forty and his mental reactions sixty, and vice-versa. The unequal functional quality of his separate organs seldom is recognized as a form of premature aging.

The man may visit his physician complaining that he is worn out at 5:00 p.m. A couple of drinks are required to pick him up. Appetite is lost. The bowels are lazy. The slightest physical effort exhausts him. He needs sleeping pills and wakes up without much desire to work. His memory is failing, and, although the libido is often present, the sexual function is far from desirable. He lives in a constant state of anxiety and joy has left his life. Even so, the most careful medical examination does not show any organic trouble or lesion.

The number of people who look, behave, and feel older than they are is increasing every day. Many start showing these signs in their twenties, and those over forty are so common that they attribute their health problems to "getting old." A good proportion of people over sixty, in view of their physical conditions, should act and appear far younger than they do, but early debilitation is accepted by them as the natural course of events. Informed people, like Ashley Montague, whose quote we used to introduce this chapter, say the trick to staying alert, active, and healthy "is very simple—die young as late as possible."[2]

It may seem paradoxical, in this age of unprecedented longevity, to speak of premature aging. The average life expectancy at birth is well over seventy years; never have so many people lived for so long. It is tempting to settle the issue by saying that premature aging is better than premature death.

But this is not the whole story. A few years ago, there appeared an intriguing appendix to the annual World Health Statistic Report, published by the (WHO) World Health Organization.[3] In it, epidemiologists and computer specialists analyzed life-expectancy statistics of thirty-four industrialized countries, dealing not only with life expectancy at birth, but life expectancy at the age of sixty-five.

The difference between the two is, of course, of great importance. Life expectancy at birth increases in a spectacular fashion when childhood diseases are effectively treated or prevented and when major infectious diseases are controlled. Life expectancy at age sixty-five gives different indications, reflecting the advance of the frontiers of longevity against the degenerative or wasting diseases. Today, these degenerative diseases are responsible for the overwhelming majority of "deaths from old age" (although there is no such thing).

The significant aspect of the WHO study is that it showed a man's life expectancy at age sixty-five being greater in such countries as Greece (79.3 years) and Iceland (80.3 years), two of the least industrialized nations of the world, than it is in the United States or in most Western European countries. (The average life expectancy for both Canadians and Americans is seventy-three years.)

Moreover, a comparison with figures recorded by WHO ten years earlier, shows that in twenty-three of the thirty-four nations included in the current study, the life expectancy of sixty-five year-old men had decreased, however slightly.

Medicine may have solved many problems regarding the

treatment or prevention of specific diseases, but it has not solved the non-specific problems of the readaptation of the human mind and organism to an increasing number of relatively sudden alterations away from natural living. These alterations lead to a certain psycho-physiology syndrome of symptoms one can label premature aging. The multiple changes in our way of life and our environment created through technology require adaptation. This demand for adaptive activity has been identified as the essence of stress.

Premature Aging from Stress

Continuous stress and tension—the condition of the modern person's life—wears out his resistance, and he becomes an easy prey to all degenerative forces. Usually, when the modern Western worker has succeeded in winning the battle for the material values of this world, he becomes incapacitated and unable to enjoy them. What good is the possibility of the prolongation of his survival, if he is denied the fundamental means to take advantage of the added years? Our society is filled with these "half-invalids" whose contribution to the community and themselves is limited by premature aging.

Stress has been the object of many recent studies and we do discuss it at length in Chapter Six. Here, we can provide one inescapable conclusion: The number of stressful events, or stressors, in modern society has been gradually increasing. These varied causative factors all produce essentially the same biologic stress response, the general adaptation syndrome, or GAS.[4]

There is little reason to doubt that stress has become a major limiting factor in the longevity of adult people. Although we know its consequences, or at least some of them, we cannot, nor shall we ever be able to, avoid stress. As Dr. Hans Selye has pointed out many times, "Complete freedom from stress is death." We must meet stress, learn how to cope with it, and attempt to limit its deleterious effects.

The way to overcome constant exposure to stressors is to supply our bodies and minds with optimal nutrition and our normal complement of exercise. Failing this, we must then emphasize the role of cognitive process as a major intermediary against many stressors. Your attitude toward life, your behavioral code, your lifestyle, in short, your whole personal philosophy, is an essential mediator in the reaction to a stressful situation.

So-called "functional patients" are not well understood by physicians who hesitate to become involved in the personal problems that may be the key to a pathologic condition. Even if the psychic origin of a disease is recognized, the use of psychotropic drugs is often resorted to, rather than an attempt at understanding and eliminating the imbalance that is the origin of the trouble.

The patient has come to expect drugs, surgery or radiation therapy, which can be helpful indeed, but which often fail to reach the crux of the problem. Certainly, none of these is corrective for the premature aging. Even if the physician takes the time to delve into the personality and the psychic problems of his patient, his authority in this field is unclear, and recommendations concerning behavior modifications are notoriously less acceptable than drug prescriptions.

Nevertheless, and in spite of the frustrations it involves, the search for psychic equilibrium is an important part of the therapeutic process. In our experience, understanding of the patient (even if it is never complete) can help the patient help himself. This is particularly true of the "functional" patient, or one suffering from degenerative diseases that precipitate premature aging in a society where healthy longevity should be unparalleled in history.

Until biologists and gerontologists discover the "aging factor," no miraculous elixir will prevent the normal aging process or premature aging. On the other hand, it is commonly observed that many people look, feel, and behave far younger than their chronological age indicates. This is achieved by a continuous and careful discipline, involving orthomolecular nutrition, an optimal diet, and exercise. This is the way to slow down the aging process—and since the process is often precipitated by psychosomatic stress, the psyche is a good place to start. This is true psychosomatic and holistic medicine. (It cannot be holistic if it is not psychosomatic.)

The Diagnoses of Pseudosenility

Senility is not psychosomatic, although the presence of senility is not a definitive diagnosis. The condition is a syndrome which appears in the aging and aged for a variety of reasons. In each case, an attempt is mandatory to determine the reason for the senility and if it is treatable. Otherwise treatment must be directed at easing the syndrome of disabling symptoms.

"Senility is one of the most serious medical diagnoses that can be given to a patient because the prognosis is so serious and the effectiveness of treatment is not clear," says Leslie Libow, M.D., chief of geriatric medicine at the Jewish Institute for Geriatric Care in New Hyde Park, New York. "If we value our older people, how can anyone seriously argue that every physcan should not do the tests to make sure a treatable cause has not been overlooked?"[5]

Any deteriorating lesion in the brain, whether biochemical or anatomical, will produce a senile-like syndrome—a pseudosenility. Treatable diseases of the brain are divided into two groups: (1) the types where there is no known anatomical pathology such as an embolism, hemorrhage, or thrombus and (2) the known problems present either as a cause or as a complication. In the discussion that follows on the occurrence of pseudosenility, the organic causes of senile-like symptoms such as the brain tumors and the rare lipid diseases of the brain are not considered.

Pseudosenility Disease Groups with No Organic Pathology

Depression which occurs in a young or middle-aged person isn't confused with senility because of the invariant tie-in of senility with old age. In differentiating a diagnosis, the myth of this irrelevant equation serves a useful purpose. However, depression does happen commonly in a senile person, and the two problems will be combined. The senility, in fact, may mimic depression so faithfully that the latter will be missed altogether.

Whether there is an apparent psychosocial reason for the presence of depression or not, it must be suspected. A patient prone to depression in the past will have a greater probability for it now. Depression comes on relatively fast with a lot of complicating irritability attached. Insomnia may also appear.

A substantial number of people are walking around with mild schizophrenia and able to maintain themselves in the community. Often they are considered slightly odd by neighbors and accepted as eccentrics. As they grow older, unfortunately, these eccentricities tend to worsen. The twin insult of the schizophrenia and aging may bring on a senile form of schizophrenia which is difficult to distinguish from outright senility. Schizophrenia in the aged is, therefore, mislabeled as senility when it's a pseudosenile set of circumstances.

The test is whether schizophrenia was present at any time in the person's past. Also, since a family history of it increases the probability of the patient's condition, the presence of schizophrenia in first-order relatives is another main diagnostic determinant. It won't be difficult to diagnose the problem of an aged, chronic schizophrenic, but even here symptoms of senility will be intertwined with the symptoms of schizophrenia.

Any history of prolonged malnutrition, especially when combined with severe stress, should throw suspicion on nutritional dependency as a cause of pseudosenility. It may change to true senility from chronic malnourishment even with the intake of large amounts of food. It's really the quality of food that counts. The most common nutritional dependency is vitamin B-3.

We believe most people who become truly senile suffer from many decades of mild to moderate malnutrition, from excessive consumption of food artifacts. A *food artifact* is a component extracted from agricultural produce as a source of raw material and recombined into food the technologists can persuade the public to like, buy, and eat. It has very little nourishment value and is a prime cause of obesity in the United States, since a food artifact generally offers only calories. You have to eat a lot of it to get any nourishment.

Pseudosenility Disease Groups with Organic Pathology

At autopsy, some apparently senile patients have shown no or little visible brain pathology, while other elderly people with a great deal of post mortem pathology showed no senile symptoms before they died. Expanding lesions in the brain such as hemorrhages, clots, infections, tumors, and other pathology clearly evident from present behavior must receive the appropriate treatment. To depend only on vitamins, minerals, and orthomolecular nutrition would be the wrong medical care. But methods should be employed alongside specific medical treatment to improve the quality of the patients' recovery.

Some years ago, Merna Harrington, a woman suffering from a moderate cerebral hemorrhage, was given good immediate and later rehabilitative treatment. Over time, she regained most of her normal brain function. One residual symptom did not clear entirely, however, and after two years, it led her into a serious depression. She also suffered from "blocking," a series of interruptions in her logical thinking. The symptoms included an inability to remember, read, or understand very easily. Mrs. Harrington recognized her reasoning inability and memory lack and worried about them, but her complaints over these handicaps were responded to by her doctors with the words: "You'll have to live with them." She assumed correctly that this meant her physicians would never be able to help her.

She was referred for orthomolecular psychiatric care partly because of her depression and also because she was such a complainer. The woman refused to accept her previous doctor's prognosis. During our first session, she said the verdict that she would have to live with "blocking" seemed like a death sentence. "If I am forced to go on with this mental disability, I would sooner die," she declared.

Merna Harrington was started on 3 grams of nicotinic acid (vitamin B-3) and 3 grams of ascorbic acid (vitamin C) each day. Within three months, most of her disability was gone. It had cleared enough so that she could think clearly, remember recent events with no difficulty, perform her routine daily chores, and live comfortably. While these two vitamins could not have restored dead neurons, they did improve the efficiency of the undamaged portion of the woman's brain. It was able to compensate more effectively with the brain cells that remained. Her depression disappeared as well, so that today she thinks and emotes in a normal way as long as she continues with her orthomolecular nutrition.

There are diseases which are metabolic in a classical sense, or they are due to hormonal imbalances. Conditions such as Addison's disease, lipodystrophies, and hypothyroidism are included among them.

Subclinical hypothyroidism is occurring more frequently than one might imagine. It may be diagnosed early by applying the Barnes technique of measuring surface body temperature under the armpit. A reading below 97.8°F (36.0°C) when the thermometer is kept in place for ten minutes indicates subclinical hypothyroidism. A better description would be "sublaboratory" hypothyroidism since the usual laboratory tests are not sensitive enough to pick up every case. The diagnosis is confirmed by the clinical response to small amounts of thyroid extract given over several months. We suspect that many senile people suffer from sublaboratory hypothyroidism. Every elderly person who complains of feeling cold all the time, of being chilled easily, should be investigated for thyroid function. It is obvious that nutrition alone cannot repair dysfunction caused by hormone imbalances.

The Hazards of Getting Old

Dr. Frederick Zeman, who was one of the founders of geriatric medicine in the United States, said: "Disease in old age is characterized by chronicity, multiplicity, and duplicity."

Chronicity and multiplicity, alone or in tandem, won't necessarily create special problems except in terms of the patients' comfort—unless the underlying diseases are not only multiple but serious, in which case, they add to the hazards of getting old. Duplicity is the main problem. The family, friends, and physicians who are interested in the elderly person's welfare may be fooled by the pseudosenile symptoms. Communication with the patient will be far from accurate and reliable if he or she is suffering from diminished perceptual faculties—hearing, sight, attention —damaged by the impoverishment of living alone or with a partner who is similarly impaired.

Moreover, just as the immune system is not fully

developed in the newborn, it is often damaged in the presenescent. Even an accurate diagnosis may be difficult to bolster with treatment. Faltering defenses of the body may be at fault.

The elderly person's ability to withstand stress—such as severe environmental alteration, whether endogenous or exogenous—is decreased. In Chapter Seven, we will describe the stress-induced senility that took over the mind of the mother-in-law of Dr. Morton Walker.

As we mentioned in the last section, subtle or overt depression closely associated with senility can make the individual insensitive to those bodily cues that alert us to the fact that something is going wrong. The symptoms of depression such as losing weight, lethargy, and weakness may actually be the symptoms of another underlying disease process, such as cancer, with the depression caused by the cancer's symptoms.

Sometimes the first step in a diagnostic procedure is to ascertain whether the depression is drug-induced. Reserpine, a drug incorporated into many other drugs for a variety of conditions, is one major culprit. The depression may disappear rapidly once the medication is withdrawn. Also, there could be a synergistic drug interaction or an inadvertent drug overdose, the result of a patient's taking similar preparations prescribed by different doctors—each unaware of the other's involvement—as well as over-the-counter remedies suggested by the corner pharmacist or friends. These possibilities increase as pseudosenility gets more ingrained. A person will be confused as to dosage times, or he may take too much of a drug that makes him "feel better" on the theory that more is better.

Another hazard of getting old is deteriorated coordination, loss of muscle strength, or osteoarthritis with involvement of the knee in particular. A misstep will cause a muscular imbalance as the eroded joint gives in and the old person topples. Osteoporosis, described in Chapter One, makes a fall more dangerous for an elderly person than for a younger one. The loss of hardness in the bone caused by calcium depletion isn't the primary problem. The real danger is the increased porosity, a loss of density in the bone matrix. When the bone twists, the connective tissues lose their cohesiveness—like a green-stick fracture in young people—and the bone of an old person breaks like a dried-out limb of a tree. An aged individual may turn awkwardly—twist a limb in the wrong direction—and the stress will be so unusual for that particular area of bone that it crumbles.

A temporary drop in blood pressure will cause a fall. The lowered blood pressure may come from changes in heart rhythm causing a quick blockage to the brain and fainting.

A feeling of dizziness among elderly patients is not rare. They will also have attacks of nausea; ringing in the ears; decrease in hearing; sudden pallor of the skin—or flushing; headache; abnormal sensations in the face, trunk, or extremities; difficulty in swallowing or in speech; double vision or any other visual disturbances; weakness in the face or hands or legs; loss of consciousness; and a loss of the power of muscle coordination.

Respiratory infection is an acute hazard of old age. The aged can't get rid of the secretions; they cough and cough but nothing comes up because they've lost expulsive power. The secretions pile up and it becomes a matter of slow drowning.

Furthermore, secretions tend to thicken because dehydration is so often a part of the picture. And if the old person has ischemic heart disease—a condition that tends to develop in the presence of chronic obstructive pulmonary disease—pulmonary congestion interferes with lung mechanics. It predisposes to an inability to breathe. Fever and pneumonia may set in quickly. Pulmonary embolism is always a danger, particularly in senile patients who are immobilized—especially after a leg or pelvic fracture. It is also a danger to those who tend not to exercise.

Tuberculosis can be the killer of the elderly. It can come on as the result of a lesion that developed in earlier years and has gone undetected until it breaks down in later years.

Abdominal problems such as gallstones, intestinal obstructions, stress ulcers, and cancer are frequently main hazards of getting old. Others are leg ulcers, electrolyte imbalance, heart disease, bladder malfunction or enlarged prostate.

Many of these maladies can be responsible for the mental symptoms of so-called "senility." In fact, we have implied that the greatest hazards of getting old is pseudosenility, being branded as senile when you are not. For example, an elderly woman was misdiagnosed as a case of senile agitation on the basis of her wandering around the house during the night. She had been hospitalized earlier for heart disease and the wandering began as soon as she returned to her daughter's home. Her final diagnosis was simply *orthopnea*, a sense of discomfort when breathing in any but the erect sitting or standing position. The old lady was getting up in order to catch her breath. With a change in medical treatment and an improved diet using orthomolecular nutrition, both the nocturnal wandering and the mild confusion that had accompanied it disappeared. Pseudosenility had almost marked her as mentally defective for the rest of her life.

Another elderly woman who had what appeared to be senile confusion underwent a medical work-up. It revealed a blood hemoglobin of 10.5 (normal blood hemoglobin for women is 12 to 15 grams per milliliter), mildly elevated blood pressure, some hardening of the arteries, and some degree of chronic obstructive pulmonary disease. Once she was given treatment to clear up her respiratory function and enough mineral supplementation (especially iron) to push her blood hemoglobin count up to 11.5, her confusion cleared, her thinking improved and hospitalization for senility was avoided.

Finally, a seventy-eight-year-old man was diagnosed as suffering from senility on the basis of extreme confusion. He was hospitalized for mental illness. Fortunately, the old man had a daughter who was genuinely interested in him. She explained that there had been a gradual deterioration over the past year or so which pointed to senility. But on the second day of his hospitalization, his laboratory test results were reported. He had a high blood urea nitrogen reading and a urologist was called in as a consultant. The urologist found the man had an enlarged prostate and considerable bladder obstruction. The patient was sent for surgery and, once that had been done, his bladder function improved considerably, his urine output increased significantly, and his blood urea nitrogen went down to near normal levels. Startlingly, the overwhelming part of his confusion cleared, and he no longer acted senile.

His daughter was astonished. Her father hadn't been that alert and clear thinking for the prior two years. What was thought to be senility was mostly toxemia from nitrogen retention. His body and brain were being poisoned by his own urine and a pseudosenile condition had set in. The old gentleman then returned to his daughter's home, and six years later, he died there peacefully at the age of eighty-four with no mental deterioration. Had the diagnosis been left as senile brain disease, he would have been sent to a state hospital and would have died there six years earlier of kidney disease—probably with no one ever realizing what the problem was.

In elderly people, the combination of organ dysfunction and malnutrition can produce the appearance of senile confusion when it actually is pseudosenility. Yet, if a patient of fifty-five showed up with that picture, he'd be given a good medical work-up and the underlying causes would be detected and corrected. If the patient is in his seventies or older, it is all too easy to accept the symptoms of senility at face value and opt for institutionalization because the condition has been labeled "irreversible." This is another one of the hazards of getting old.

The late Massachusetts physician, Alfred Worcester, wrote:

> The aged, as we must never forget, are always lonesome. They have outlived the preceding, and very likely their own, generation; or, if any survive, only by extra good fortune can there be any more meetings. Their family separations too often have caused the additional loss of their old homes and former neighbors. To the ways and manners of the present, they are not accustomed. They belong to the unforgiving past. They are as strangers in the land.

In the next chapter, we will learn that our society is creating a land full of strangers not only among the very old but also in the earlier generations. It comes from a form of malnutrition foisted slyly on us by commercial interests because we are mostly ignorant in the ways of good eating. What's the result? Symptoms that resemble senility, caused by malnutrition.

References for Chapter Two

1. Retirement by senility. *The New York Times*, May 8, 1977.

2. Goleman, Daniel. Don't be adultish! *Psychology Today* 11:46-50, August 1977.

3. World Health Organization. *World Health Statistics Report* 25:430-442, 1972.

4. Selye, Hans. *Journal of the International Academy of Preventive Medicine* II:1-21, 1975.

5. Altman, Lawrence K. Senility is not always what it seems to be. *The New York Times*, May 8, 1977.

3

HYPOTHESES OF
SENILE PATHOLOGY

*There are no diseases of the aged, but simply diseases
among the aged.*
— Leonard Larson, M.D., President-
elect of the American Medical Association, June 27, 1960

No Senility for Remarkable Historical Figures

DURING THE GOLDEN AGE of Greece when the average
life expectancy of Greek citizens was little more than
eighteen years, reflecting the fact that most people died
at birth or in infancy, Pericles delivered his Funeral Ora-
tion, the foundation of modern democratic thought, at the
age of sixty-nine.

Charlemagne ruled until A.D. 813, and handed over the
reins of power to his son when he was seventy-one at a
time when people lived an average of just twenty-two years.

Michelangelo executed the "Pieta" when he was eighty
years old, while the average Italian life expectancy was
only to age thirty-two.

Goethe was eighty-four when Part II of "Faust" was first
published.

Disraeli did not become Britain's Prime Minister until he
was seventy, a time when the average Englishman's life
span was forty-seven years.

Sir Winston Churchill was sixty-five years old in 1939 at

the beginning of the Second World War when he led his people to victory over tyranny. He died January 24, 1965, at the age of eighty-nine.

There was no senility for the remarkable figures of history. And the antisenility roll call continues inexorably with the names of Kant, Voltaire, Titian, Khrushchev, Mao Tse-tung, Truman, Tito, de Gaulle, Queen Elizabeth I, Queen Victoria, Liszt, Plato, Einstein, Buddha, Confucius, Galileo, Copernicus, Archimedes, Edison, and John D. Rockefeller. Genghis Kahn continued to rule for seven years past our current usual age of retirement. Eisenhower was sixty-seven when he composed the "Eisenhower Doctrine."[1]

The two possible common factors that allowed for continued normal brain function for these historical figures were the inheritance of good genes and the provision of an optimal internal environment. Physicians usually do include these two factors when discussing longevity in general and an alert geriatric mind in particular. People who are concerned realize that inheritance plays a role, but there is no way of changing our genes for the better. Since genes require a suitable environment for their expression, we can try to provide an optimum environment so that even the weakest genes will serve us much better. If one's parents have lived long healthy lives, we can aspire to the same by living in such a way as to avoid the known risk factors. If our parents have been shortlived and ill, we can improve on their lifestyle by providing our cells with an optimum biochemical and physiological environment.

Of the remarkable historical figures we have named, Sir Winston Churchill is typical of a person who inherited better genes than the physiological environment in which he sheltered them. His obesity, cigar-smoking and high consumption of alcohol kept him in a relative hypoglycemic condition, and it is thought that hypoglycemic adults are more vulnerable to brain damage. He suffered a number of small strokes which left him more and more incapacitated as he approached death. It is likely that if Sir Winston had followed a healthier lifestyle, his genes would have had him living well past his hundredth year with an active and creative mind.

Our Hypothesis on the Development of Senility

Churchill's physical and possibly mental deterioration also represent the classic illustration of a working hypothesis we've developed on the cellular cause of senility. According to this hypothesis, *senility is a state of neuron inactivity brought on by anaerobic respiration of the cells*. If aerobic respiration is maintained at its optimum level, no one will become senile. This means that uninterrupted oxygen must be carried to the brain cells by a viable blood supply, that all the respiratory enzymes must remain intact, and that there is always an adequate amount of glucose in the brain with no accumulation of anaerobic metabolites. In brief, senescence is quiescence of the brain's built-in health system.

In developing this hypothesis on the pathology of senility, we were confronted with what appeared to be an insoluble problem. We examined the known facts from every angle and considered other hypotheses that exist. Now, when scientists develop a hypothesis, it is not done as an end in itself. Their function is to direct research. It is more exciting for the scientists to be proven right, but even the destruction of a hypothesis will have been valuable if the research was done well. Any hypothesis must be grounded in observations which are relevant to the problem. The odds against the hypothesis being proved right are so low that one must not indulge in flights of fancy where the odds are even lower.

Consequently, we made a number of observations which we used to develop our hypothesis regarding senility. First, we saw the effect reported by Edwin Boyle, Jr., M.D., research director of the Miami Heart Institute, where hyperbaric oxygen temporarily removed senility, as described in Chapter One. Second, we knew that the lack of oxygen (called *anaerobic*) had the effect of causing cancer. These two ideas, among others, we combined to produce the hypothesis stated above.

Otto Heinrich Warburg, one of the world's foremost biochemists, won his Nobel Prize because of basic work with respiratory enzymes and cellular mechanisms. He discovered and characterized the pyridine nucleotide dehydrogenases and flavoproteins as members of the respiratory chain, and worked out the mechanism whereby the energy released in the oxidation of foodstuffs may be conserved and transferred for use in synthesis and growth. The mechanism of cellular respiration provided the first explanation of the chemical mechanism of enzyme action.

Several years before he died, Dr. Warburg published a review of the problem of cancer. He had shown that there was a relationship between anaerobic respiration and cancer growth. When ordinary cells in pure culture are forced to live in an atmosphere which does not have enough oxygen, they switch their respiratory mechanism from one depending upon oxygen (called *aerobic*), to one not dependent upon oxygen. This change is apparently irreversible.

Even more important, the anaerobic cells begin to divide. They are no longer subject to the usual growth controls and eventually become cancerous.

Warburg also explained that the malignancy of cancer tissue was correlated with the degree of anaerobic conditions. The less oxygen there was available to the tissue, the more rapid was its growth. Rapidly growing tissues are generally more malignant than slow growing cancers.

Szent-Györgyi (1974), the discoverer of vitamin C, considered that the cancerous state is a reversal to a more primitive state of the cell.[2] This occurs because electron flow along protein molecules breaks down and not enough energy is left for the cell to keep division from taking place. In order to remain alive, the cell reverts to an anaerobic form of respiration. It can live in very low oxygen tension, where nontransformed cells would soon die.

Laki and Ladik (1976) reviewed Szent-Györgyi's work and other evidence such as that neuroblastoma cells grown rapidly in serum require little oxygen. When serum is withheld, growth stops and oxygen consumption increases. They supported Szent-Györgyi's work.[3]

Furthermore, there is an increase in acetylcholine esterase and in Krebs cycle enzymes, according to the Laki and Ladik findings. Low oxygen uptake may be due to less efficient binding of nicotinamide-adenine dinucleotide (NAD) made in the body from vitamin B-3. Addition of NAD enhances oxidative respiration.

So convinced was Dr. Warburg by his investigations of respiratory enzymes and their mechanisms, that he recommended preventive treatment measures to preclude the development of cancer. This included doing everything possible to ensure optimum aerobic conditions in the cells and the tissues. He suggested that everyone ensure optimum oxygen-carrying capacity by keeping hemoglobin levels normal. He also suggested that everyone ensure optimum levels of oxygen-carrying co-enzymes such as riboflavin, thiamin, and niacin—all B vitamins. He pointed out that a precancerous condition of the throat known as *leukoplakia* would not become cancerous if the patients were given vitamin B-3 (niacin).

The most interesting part of Warburg's report was his theory of dedifferentiation. By *dedifferentiation*, he meant the following: Evolution began with cells which lived without oxygen, in an anaerobic environment. Only later on, did enough oxygen accumulate in our atmosphere to allow cells to develop aerobic respiration. This condition is much more efficient in converting food into energy. More energy is released per gram of food in the presence of oxygen. It is likely that multicellular organisms did not develop until cells became aerobic. While single-celled species had only one function—to divide—multi-celled organisms demanded that other functions live together in harmony. Anaerobic respiration is associated with cell division as the main function. Aerobic respiration permits growth as well as other cellular functions. According to Warburg's theory, the switch back from aerobic to anaerobic respiration brings back the primitive cell division as the only function of the cell, something he labeled *dedifferentiation*.

This dedifferentiation can only bring on uncontrolled cell division among those cells still retaining the ability to divide.

What would happen to cells not able to divide, such as neurons? A baby is born with its full complement of neurons. Thereafter, they are lost at a slow pace daily until the individual dies. Neurons never regenerate, as pointed out in Chapter One.

The inability to regenerate exists because each neuron had a large number of dendrites and long nerves. It is impossible to conceive how such a cell could divide and produce two cells, each with the proper attachments to other cells. There are no neuron cancers. Neurons cannot divide. Therefore, dedifferentiation of neurons cannot cause cancer. In other words, anaerobic respiration of neurons won't cause cancer. Then what happens? Since the neurons in the cortex are no longer able to carry on their main function and don't divide, they simply become quiescent. The result is senility. This is our hypothesis—*senescence is neuron quiescence*.

Other Hypotheses of Senile Pathology

In 1977, Dr. R. E. Myers reported that the actual cause of damage to the brain when the blood circulation is shut off is the accumulation of lactic acid; it is not strictly caused from the lack of oxygen. In an experiment he performed, monkeys were not given any food for twenty-four hours and then their ability to withstand a stoppage in blood flow for 12-14 minutes was tested. No detectable damage in the animals was found. Even after twenty-four minutes, the neurologic findings were minimal. Next, the researcher infused glucose into another group of monkeys before causing a new circulatory arrest, and this produced a different picture. After fourteen minutes, the animals developed irreversible changes so that they had to be killed, or they died. Chemical analyses showed that these monkey brains had ten times as much lactate in the animals fed glucose as compared to a mere four-fold increase in the food-deprived animals.[4]

Although this work has not yet been applied to people, it should be. The experiments done by Myers indicate that blood glucose levels should remain at the fasting level, or as close to it as possible, for everyone who wants to avoid senile pathology. This may be achieved by avoiding all free sugar by the use of a hypoglycemic diet. Taking note again of Sir Winston Churchill's condition, it now seems likely that people who avoid sugar in their diet may have fewer strokes, and if they do have one, will stand a much better chance of surviving it with their brain intact. The trick is to avoid processed sugar of any kind.

Furthermore, this also means that the hospital administration of glucose solutions should be given with great care and very slowly, or not at all, to anyone at risk. Myers concludes,

> These findings direct our attention to a greater concern with the rationale for administering glucose to women in labor—especially those cases where the risk of fetal asphyxia is high. These findings are also relevant to the management of critically ill newborns suffering from respiratory problems and experiencing episodes of apnea.

(*Apnea* is the absence of breathing.)

Women in labor should receive snacks of whole food such as seeds, nuts, fresh vegetables and yogurt. They should not be fed any food artifact whatever such as refined carbohydrate like cake, candy, Jello, and cola drinks. Depriving the mother-to-be of a processed sugared product might decrease the incidence of infant cerebral damage from lack of oxygen. This anoxia is one of the causes of infant learning disorders and a child's hyperactive behavior. Hypoglycemic women are likely to have a greater incidence of disturbed infants, and hypoglycemic adults are more vulnerable to senile brain damage for the same reason.

Accordingly, senility is a state of neuron inactivity caused by anaerobic respiration of the cells. The cells' ability to become active is still there and can be reactivated by increasing the amount of oxygen available as with hyperbaric oxygen. So far, however, medical scientists have no way of permanently maintaining aerobic respiration. Prolonged hyperbaric oxygen would be dangerous, because it tends to increase the free radical concentration. This has pernicious effects leading to premature aging and eventual senility, the very problems we are attempting to avoid. The problem is to provide optimal amounts of oxygen to allow proper aerobic respiration and to protect the body against the oxidative potential of oxygen and free radicals. Any comprehensive anti-senility program must take all these factors into account.

Accepting the working hypothesis put forth earlier, that senility is dedifferentiation caused by a conversion of aerobic to anaerobic respiration, it follows that any process which reduces the delivery of oxygen to the brain cells, or prevents its utilization, will hasten senility. These factors include lack of oxygen in the inhaled air, anemia, circulatory difficulty, and a deficiency of respiratory enzymes in the brain. The most common exposure to decreased atmospheric oxygen occurs during airplane flights. Presenile people ought not to be exposed to decreased oxygen pressure in aircraft cabins for long periods of time.

Another problem is the red blood cells' affinity for adherence to each other—*the rouleoux effect*. When red blood cells stick to each other, like stacked coins in a bank's coin roll, the blood is prevented from flowing freely into the capillaries. Single red blood cells travel through capillaries delivering the oxygen to surrounding cells. A group of cells are unable to enter. At bifurcations of vessels, there will be an uneven distribution of cells. One vessel may carry a lot of plasma with few cells, while another may carry too many clumped cells. In either case, not enough oxygen is delivered—called sludging.

Sludging may be seen readily by looking into the eye with a slit lamp. Small blood vessels there possess no red cells in them. People with marked sludging have certain clinical characteristics. Their faces are pale and puffy due to swelling; their eyes are not alert; they suffer from fatigue, tension and anxiety. A large number of middle-aged and elderly people have this characteristic clinical syndrome. When they are treated with nicotinic acid, they regain their normal facial appearance and color. Dr. Edwin Boyle observed that nicotinic acid restored the normal homogeneous nature of the blood. The red blood cells once more repelled each other, probably by increasing the electronegative charge on each cell.

Walsh, Melaney and Walsh (1977) also believe that sludging is a major factor in causing senility. Conditions which bring on sludging such as diabetes and alchoholism accelerate the senile symptoms. Moreover, they found that treatment with anticoagulants which are antisludging medications were useful in retarding senility.[5] Walsh and Walsh treated forty-nine seniles with the anticoagulant Coumadin. Of this group, 70 percent improved—15 percent dramatically. Walsh had given another anticoagulant, Decumarol, to twenty-four seniles in 1968 with even better results. Even though Decumarol is more difficult to use clinically, because it produces more side effects, it appears to give a better result.[6]

Of the other biochemical hypotheses fashioned to explain aging and senility, we consider the cross linkage theory proposed by Bjornksten (1960-1971), to be among the most promising.[7,8,9,10,11] It is a highly technical explanation of the senile's pathology, and we will try to present it as simply as possible. Bjornksten and his collaborators suggested that certain metabolites of molecules in the body, arising from excessive oxidation, combine with two or more long protein molecules to bind them together. An unnatural cross link forms. The cross-linked protein no longer is able to function normally and can't be split or hydrolized by enzymes usually present in the body.

This cross-linking is analogous to the vulcanization of rubber. Here, long rubber molecules which float free in solution are bound to each other by other short molecules to form the familiar rubber substance. It is elastic, tough, and can no longer be dealt with by natural enzymes. The same kind of vulcanization effect appears to take place in elderly skin. This largest organ of the body becomes inelastic, brittle, and parchment-like. It is easy to visualize the similarity of senile skin and aged or oxidized rubber. With deteriorated rubber, the process of cross linkage production of oxidation has gone too far.

The excessive formation of small molecules which can form cross linkages is the real villain. These highly reactive molecules include quinones, chrome indoles such as dopachrome, noradrenochrome and adrenochrome, aldehydes and oxidizing ions such as copper. Such substances are synthesized in greater quantity by exposure to radiation, to smoking, and to excessive oxygen, or by disease such as diabetes mellitus. Too much copper in the body and a deficiency of zinc will do the same. Perhaps all the toxic heavy metals also do the same, including lead, cadmium, aluminum, mercury, silver and gold.

Playing another part in senile pathology must be the long protein molecule which undergoes certain changes to make reactive groups more available for cross linkage.

Molecules folded into certain configurations may be less apt to be cross-linked.

Evidence that free radicals are involved in aging was contributed by Harman (1956, 1962).[12,13] The free radicals are highly reactive molecules half-way between an oxidized and reduced state. These are especially apt to occur in plasma which is rich in oxygen and in oxidizing enzymes including ceruloplasmin, the copper-rich enzyme, and hemoglobin.

Cross linkage would be particularly injurious in certain tissues such as in blood vessel walls. Cross linkage would shorten protein chains, make them inelastic or brittle, and increasingly subject them to failure. Blood vessels must be able to expand and contract in harmony with the heat of the heart, but cross linkage would not permit that. Also, the cross-linked vessel wall would be less permeable to the transfer of essential nutrients to the cells.

Harman and Piette (1966) found direct evidence that oxygen increased free radical formation in blood from the natural substrates adrenalin and noradrenalin.[14]

Bjornksten (1968, 1971) aptly summarized the current cross linkage theory:

> Crosslinking is damaging to the tissues and involves loss of elasticity, reduced swelling capacity, increased resistance to hydrolases and probably enzymes generally, and thus an increase in molecular weight and a tendency toward embrittlement. There is a growing amount of direct evidence and much indirect evidence for postulating the relationship between crosslinking and aging.[15,16]
>
> Crosslinking agents present in the living organism include aldehydes, lipid oxidation products, sulfur alkylating agents, quinones, free radicals induced by ionizing radiation, antibodies, polybasic acids, polyhalo derivatives and polyvalent metals. The latter four types of compound are slow-acting but can also ac-

cumulate in the body to form a frozen metabolic pool. Sufficient amounts of all these potential cross-linking materials are present in the body to make the changes of aging unavoidable.

Bullough (1973) suggested that stress could delay death by its effect on tissue chalones. A *chalone* is a tissue specific antimitotic messenger molecule present in all mammalian tissues. The antimitotic power of chalones is increased by adrenaline and by a glucocorticord hormone. This is why cells divide more rapidly during sleep when adrenalin secretion is lower. Bullough postulates that the chalones not only inhibit mitosis (cell division) but also retard aging. In other words, chalones retard senility by combining these two reactions. In tissues which do not divide (neurons), the mitotic process is permanently switched off early in life, and these cells live much longer. By age seventy, however, about 10 percent of all the neurons present at birth have been lost.[17]

Adrenaline is easily oxidized by adrenochrome in the test tube and probably in the body, as well. The evidence is summarized in *The Hallucinogens* by Hoffer and Osmond (1967).[18] Adrenochrome is one of the most potent mitotic poisons, for it stops cells from dividing. Most likely the antimitotic properties of adrenaline arise from its conversion into adrenochrome. Adrenochrome is in turn converted into two classes of indoles, a dihydroxy series which is nontoxic and may have antistress properties, and a trihydroxy series (adrenalutin) which is toxic in a different way than adrenochrome. Production of adrenochrome requires oxygen. Anoxia, which leads to anaerobic respiration, would shut off the production of adrenochrome and its antimitotic effect. Is this why anaerobic respiration increases cell division to favor cancer?

Bullough made another interesting suggestion. He pointed out that when a number of different tissues must work together, it is usual for one tissue to act as initiator and pacemaker. If aging is dictated by deterioration of non-mitotic tissue, then, he suggests, one of these tissues may play the leading role. The three nondividing tissues are neurons and muscle cells in heart, and muscle cells in other muscles. The brain must be the initiator and pace-maker of these three. Nervous deterioration does lead to muscular deterioration and in turn deterioration of the circulation.

The Summary of Senile Pathology Hypotheses

In summary, most of the theories of aging and senility involve oxidation. These are: (1) the cross linkage theory with its free radical theory; (2) Bullough's tissue chalone hypothesis; (3) Myers's work on anoxia and lactic acid accumulation; (4) the Warburg and Szent-Györgyi hypoth-esis on cancer; and (5) the work relating senility to hyperbaric oxygen researched by Boyle.

The basic biological problem appears to be to provide optimum amounts of oxygen for oxidation. Too little may lead to cancer in mitotic tissues, and to senility in nonmitotic neurons. Too much oxygen leads to physical senility by accelerating free radical formation and cross linkage for-mation.

Programs designed to prevent senility should seek to avoid cross-linking. This may be done by preventing the formation of additional cross linkages, by breaking up those already formed, and by eliminating protein mole-cules already hopelessly cross-linked. A consistent scheme would include:

1. Reduce the formation of free radicals:
   i. Avoid radiation, cigarette smoke, excessive oxygena-tion, excessive copper and other toxic elements.
   ii. Increase availability of antioxidants such as ascorbic

acid (vitamin C), alpha tocopherol (vitamin E), and ensure enough zinc, selenium and other antioxidant elements.

2. Decrease the tendency of protein molecules to be cross-linked. There is no information upon which we can call to accomplish this, and the only way so far is to decrease formation of free radicals.

3. Eliminate aged protein molecules. Bjornksten is looking for enzymes or other methods for breaking cross-linked molecules into smaller molecules which are easier to eliminate.

We suspect that one of the main functions of skin and its appendages, hair and nails, is to excrete cross-linked proteins. It is a property of the body to deposit in the skin large molecules which cannot be excreted in the feces or in urine. Human skin grows and wears away, taking with it whatever has been deposited, in the same way that trees get rid of accumulations of minerals by shedding their leaves. The skin is a protein structure, obviously cross-linked, since it is tough but resilient and elastic. It contains more free radicals when exposed to sun and radiation. The result of free radical activity is obvious, and everyone has seen it on themselves or on others. A suntan is the result of free radical action on molecules such as dopa and other amines.

We have seen increased melanin formation in patients receiving nicotinic acid—a few schizophrenics on the vitamin notice that their skin, especially on the flexor surfaces (under armpit, wrist, and on inner aspect of elbow), will turn dark brown. There is more melanin there. However, this is a benign change and after a while, no longer occurs. The pigmented skin wears away leaving healthy, normally pigmented skin. This can be accelerated by rubbing the wet skin gently. The pigment will rub off easily, much as does an old suntan. The excess free radicals seem to be deposited in the skin for excretion by the skin. We have seen similar changes in the nails. Perhaps the excessive pigmentation in pellagra is an attempt by the body to get rid of unusually high amounts of free radicals. Perhaps some cross-linked proteins are also deposited in skin to be eliminated.

References for Chapter Three

1. Calvert, Pamela. Senility roll call. Letters to the editor of *The New York Times*, October 14, 1977.

2. Szent-Györgyi, A. *Life Sciences* 15:863, 1974.

3. Laki, K. and Ladik, J. A note on the "electronic theory" of cancer. *International Journal of Quantum Chemistry* 3: 51-57, 1976.

4. Myers, R. E. Report to the Second Joint Stroke Conference. Reported in *Medical Post*, Toronto, March 29, 1977.

5. Walsh, A.C.; Melaney, C.; and Walsh, B. Paper presented to the American Psychiatric Association meeting in Toronto, 1977.

6. Walsh, A.C. and Walsh, B.H. Presenile dementia: further experience with an anti-coagulant psychotherapy regimen. *Journal of the American Geriatrics Society* 22:467-472, 1974.

7. Bjorksten, J. A common denominator in aging research. *Texas Reports on Biology and Medicine* 18: 347-357, 1960.

8. Bjorksten, J. Aging primary mechanism. *Gerontologia* 8:179-192, 1963.

9. Bjorksten, J. Chemical causes of the aging process. *Procedures of the Scientific Section of the Toilet Goods Association* 41:32-34, 1964.

10. Bjorksten, J. The crosslinkage theory of aging. *Journal of the American Geriatrics Society* 16:408-427, 1968.

11. Bjorksten, J. The crosslinkage theory of aging. *Finska Kemists Meds* 80:23-38, 1971.

12. Harman, D. Aging: a theory based on free radical and radiation chemistry. *Journal of Gerontology* 11:298-300, 1956.

13. Harman, D. Role of free radicals in mutation, cancer, aging, and maintenance of life. *Radiation Research* 16:753-763, 1962.

14. Harman, D. and Piette, L. H. Free radical theory of aging: free radical reactions in serum. *Journal of Gerontology* 21:560-565, 1966.

15. Bjorksten, J. The crosslinkage theory of aging. *Journal of the American Geriatrics Society* 16:408-427, 1968.

16. Bjorksten, J. The crosslinkage theory of aging. *Finska Kemists Meds* 80:23-38, 1971.

17. Bullough, W. S. Aging of mammals. (*Zeit fur alternsforchung*) 27, 247-253, 1973.

18. Hoffer, A. and Osmond, H. *The Hallucinogens.* New York: Academic Press, 1967.

SENILITY FROM SUBTLE, CHRONIC MALNUTRITION

The cells of our bodies can become unwell and malfunctioning for two general reasons: First, they may be poisoned; second, they may lack a good supply of nourishing food. This nourishing food must be a complex mixture of chemicals (water is one of these "chemicals") in about the right proportions. Included in this food must be about ten or more amino acids, about fifteen vitamins, and a similar number of minerals, all in addition to the fuel—carbohydrate and fat—that our bodies need to run on in the sense that an automobile needs gasoline. All of the food elements enter our body by way of the open mouth, and the health of all the cells of our bodies depends upon whether or not we place within our open mouths the proper kind of food.

—Roger J. Williams, Ph.D., *Nutrition Against Disease,* 1971

Nutrition Experts Urge Study of Elderly's Needs

NEARLY EVERY STUDY of aging and/or senility by physicians interested in nutrition, or by nutritionists themselves, has shown that diet plays a role.

Doctors at the National Institute on Aging conference held in Washington, D.C., June 7, 1978, recommended that the United States Government sponsor research on what diets the elderly should follow. The nutrition experts said that too little attention has been paid to the nutritional needs of the elderly, despite the fact that nutrition can play a key role in reducing diseases in old age.

Dr. Robert N. Butler, the director of the National Institute on Aging, said that our entire society stands to benefit by improving the health of the elderly. More than half of the U.S. health expenditures in 1976 went for the medical care of the 23 million Americans who are sixty-five or over.

"In old age, the composition of the body changes, with lean body mass being reduced and the proportion of fat increased," said Dr. Robert E. Shank, a professor at Washington University in St. Louis, speaking before this same conference. "The elderly usually are advised to eat less than when they were young, but they still require the same amount of nutrients."[1]

In 1949 and 1950, Stieglitz wrote that senile changes of the body were primarily due to cellular malnourishment. All the degenerative diseases share in common impairment of the nutrition of our body cells. This could be due to any one or any combination of at least four factors:

1. Inadequate supply of food with a deficiency of essential nutrients
2. Inefficient distribution because of circulatory impairment
3. Ineffective utilization due to enzyme deficiencies.
4. Accumulation of injurious metabolic debris, or as they have been called—"clinkers".

Stieglitz concluded that minor degrees of vitamin deficiencies were present in most people, and he recommended doubling the intake because "wise nutrition is a most powerful tool for the attainment of vigor in later years." What he decided was extraordinary when you consider that in 1950, the vitamin dependency concepts popular today had not yet been developed.[2,3]

We believe that his first factor, deficiency of essential

nutrients, when present for many decades in the form of subtle, chronic malnutrition, is the source of most premature aging and final senility.

We are convinced, moreover, that the operating of factor one for a long time will lead to problems in factor three, enzyme deficiencies, and later to factor four, the accumulation of undesirable products of abnormal metabolism. There will be a substantial number of people in whom factor three alone will force the average diet to be inadequate.

It is probable that elderly people who live well into old age without becoming senile have been skillful in their selection of food, or they have had digestive systems better able to extract essential nutrients from their food. Yet, in 1959, Droller and Dossett found senile patients were low in serum vitamin B-12,[4] and in 1962, Kral also found that malnutrition was a common problem of the elderly.[5] These are aspects of aging and senility which have been almost totally ignored by establishment geriatricians. Our contention is that too much money and time has been squandered in looking for psychosocial explanations for senility, and an absolutely inadequate amount has been used to explore the biochemical basis of this degenerative disease. We positively assert that senility arises from subtle, chronic malnutrition derived from the inappropriate application of food technology and the selling of the products resulting from that technology to victimized consumers.

Sophisticated but Simplistic Food Technology

It is easy to understand what good nutrition is if it is accepted as a basic rule that all animals should eat what the species has adapted to during evolution. Obviously, deer won't be healthy if forced to eat meat and wolves will die if forced to eat only grass. Other animals including man are not so exclusive and can eat various types of food, but this is merely a way of highlighting the idea that every species should consume only what it has been adapted to. It is important to understand why this is essential.

All food must be broken down in the body into its simplest components: proteins into amino acids, carbohydrates into glucose, fats into fatty acids. This process requires enzymes. If they are not present, the food will be of no value whatever to the animal. A dog's digestive tract cannot split grasses. But a ruminant, such as a cow, has a mechanism for storing these complex polysaccharides while they are fermented by microorganisms, which do the basic digestion. In the same way, termites contain in their digestive tract microorganisms which can digest wood. Even when the food can be broken down, it is still essential that the proportions of proteins, carbohydrates and fats present are the same or similar to those in the food the species has adapted to, with, of course, adequate amounts of vitamins and essential elements.

The same set of food rules applies to the nutrition of humans. It would be unlikely to persuade people to vary too far from eating substances they could not digest. We don't feed them hay as a staple, no matter how nutritious it is for horses. But today's food technology violates the common sense of good nutrition on a grand scale.

Food technology has run rampant, with no controls by nutritionists or physicians. It employs the oldest concepts of nutritional science with the newest methods of food extraction. The old nutrition classifies food in the simplest of terms—proteins, fats, and so forth—and reveals no comprehension of the relationship between cellular and molecular interactions. The old science consists in adding up the individual factors, using totally inadequate allowances such as Recommended Daily Allowances (RDA), which are absolutely meaningless for the individual organism.

On the one hand, food technology is simplistic in its approach to the science of nourishment, and on the other, it is highly sophisticated in its extraction techniques of individual food components. The result is a sophisticated but subtle form of chronic malnutrition suffered by some of the world's most affluent citizens.

Thus, the nutritional model followed now near the end of the twentieth century is still the nineteenth century model. We don't have the benefit of eating the whole foods popular in the nineteenth century, however, because modern food technology is refining away the vital wholeness of any natural food and splitting it into separate components we have labeled *artifacts*.

Another nineteenth century hangover is toxicology. Individual chemicals are tested to see if they will kill animals, or cause disease such as cancer, and if so, at what dose level. It is assumed that quantities below that toxic level are safe, but toxicologists have not been testing combinations of chemicals. Individual chemicals may well be nontoxic, while in combination, they can be quite toxic, although the quantity of each is nontoxic. Nor has anyone tested the combined effect of dozens of these chemicals added all together to our daily food. No one really knows how many chemicals are slipped into our diet. Estimates suggest that several thousand become part of the food supply, but it is probably much more.

When any chemical is synthesized or extracted, it carries with it into the final product traces of the chemicals used in its manufacture. It is not practical to produce 100 percent pure material, for its cost would be prohibitive. Any additive must therefore carry with it, even if in traces, an imprint of all the chemicals used to make it and purify it. But no one had determined the amount of these traces, nor their cumulative effect, over a period of thirty or forty years. Probably this will never be done, for scientists would need to test a manufactured food over decades using a constant procedure to ensure that the composition of the food remained invariant from the beginning to the end of the experiment.

You could feed test animals the final food which appears in packages in the store for several generations, but this is seldom done. It would be sensible if manufacturers were required to prove that any product they make is as nutritious as the raw foodstuff from which it was made, on the basis of feeding experiments and not on the basis of composition or RDAs. If their products contained only 70 percent of the nutritional value, this would be shown on the labels in large numbers. A pizza pie would list on its label the proportion of each food stuff used, such as so much cheese, so much white flour or whole wheat flour, so much sugar, and all the other ingredients plus the one evaluative figure. Then each purchaser would, at a glance, be able to compare the single convenience product with natural food.

Ross Hume Hall, Ph.D., Professor of Biochemistry at McMaster University Health Center, Ontario, Canada, points out that we need a new science of nourishment. We believe that these new scientists society is searching for are the orthomolecular physicians and nutritionists. They understand both food technology and nutrition. Our present food technologists do not understand nutrition, while our modern nutritionists don't understand how food technology has depleted the nutritional value of our food. Go to any convention of dieticians or establishment nutritionists and you'll see them gorging on assorted junk and cola drinks supplied gratis by the manufacturers to build good will and promote sales among these so-called food experts. Their behavior is hypocritical and puts the lie to anything they recommend as being healthy nutrition.

Government agencies which control industry, in turn, fall back on nineteenth century nutritional ideas so that their edicts bear no relation to the real world of modern convenience foods. The deep-fat-fried, sugared, white flour superdonut is an example of malnourishment. The donut is a mixture of the three most undesirable food artifacts: white flour, pure fat, and pure sucrose. The superdonut contains small quantities of some of the vitamins. To a person informed on matters of nutrition, it is shocking to be told that two donuts plus a glass of milk furnishes one-third of the RDA for protein and these vitamins. This has been approved in the United States for school lunch programs. As Hall puts it,

> Thus, a product filled with sugar, chemically manipulated fat, and other artificial ingredients with the wave of a vitamin wand becomes a highly nutritious breakfast. Such nutrition fakery is going to become more prominent as the FDA moves toward approval of vitamin fortification of fabricated foods in general.

The following is another example of deteriorated nourishment through technology: The FDA recently ruled that an artificial product need not be labeled artificial or imitation if its nutrient content is similar to that of the natural. The public will not know whether its orange juice comes from a tree or from a chemical factory.

Breakfast foods probably represent the worst examples of the conversion of food into food artifact—junk. A large supermarket may contain over one hundred breakfast cereals. The supermarket shopper would think this provides a splendid variety of food with which to balance the diet. But a look at the contents shows these colorful cereals are prepared from just a few grains (rice, corn, wheat), many sugars, corn syrup, synthetic colors and several chemicals as additional additives. We have, in fact, over one hundred different concoctions of flour, sugar and chemicals. Any health food store providing the grains and seeds has a much greater variety of good food, but a much smaller variety of these precooked artificial cereals. Many years ago, the word "ersatz" was used to label a coffee substitute, and it was a derogatory word. "Ersatz" should be resurrected and applied to all our modern, precooked breakfast cereals with a warning label that this ersatz product will be definitely injurious to your health.

Mankind evolved over centuries eating a variety of foods which provide certain trophic factors as well as the basic components of one's diet. Trophic factors are extra nutrients that probably come from the molecular constitution of a food, or may be due to chemicals still not identified individually as being essential. Trophic factors are removed by processing along with the wide variety of foodstuff also destroyed.

Almost 60 percent of all calories in North America come from white flour, fat and sugar—all non-nutritive products.

The enormous proliferation of what appears to be food—synthetics—would be impossible without food additives. These are chemicals that do not add any nutritional merit to food. They have made possible the modern supermarket carrying over ten thousand items made from a few processed materials. There is an infinite number of product forms, colorful, palatable, stable, easily prepared —but junk. They have no redeeming value. Without the additives, nearly all these junk products would disappear.

The combination of 1800 additives with a few processed high calorie products has never been tested biologically. The food industry is aware that people prefer what appears to be food, but actually is not. Why else would they try so hard to make synthetic foods? For preparing tomato soup, one can now buy a synthetic tomato extender which is 50 percent sugar plus synthetic coal tar derived dyes and the trace impurities present in each additive. This is recommended for making juices, soup, and other convenience items. Even simple substances such as cornstarch are chemically treated to withstand the shock of high temperature processing, and to ensure its stability. Cornstarch is no longer a natural starch. Another example is an imitation honey which appears to be identical with honey, but contains very little real honey.

Government agencies have given up trying to control the quality of food generated by industry. Professor Hall described to us a report in a Canadian newspaper that said Dr. Alex B. Morrison, Chief of Health Protection Branch of Ottawa, eats a highly nutritious natural diet. He even grinds his own wheat to make whole wheat flour. Professor Hall said:

> When it comes to making public recommendations, they fall back on scientific criteria, which in the case of nutrition and safety, are limited. They can, therefore, pronounce quite sincerely, "There's no evidence that such and such food is harmful." Nevertheless when it comes to their own personal life, they make use of their own scientific intuition and personal convictions.

The Denutrifaction of the Staff of Life

Our last example of the effect of subtle, sophisticated, chronic malnutrition from food technology will be bread—the staff of life—especially for many aged who cannot afford a variety of food or cannot chew rougher, healthier food.

Wheat is ordinarily a nutritious food. Each kernel contains everything necessary to start a new plant. Breadmaking became industrialized when one of the first assembly lines for the manufacture of ships' biscuits was begun in 1833 by the British Admiralty.

Wheat was originally made into flour, either by pounding it or grinding it between large stones. Eventually it was crushed between steel rollers which made it possible to remove bran and germ leaving a highly refined white flour.

Freshly milled flour is said to be "green" and is not mature. This means that when baked, the cells of the dough are not tough enough to retain gas and the loaf does not rise as much. It does not produce an even textured slice risen to its capacity to expand. But white flour stored several months does become mature. The oxidation gradually strengthens the protein walls of the gas cells, and the yellow carotene converted into vitamin A in the body is bleached, producing a pure white slice.

A mill which might make 10,000, one hundred pound packs of flour a day would require enormous warehouse space to age the flour. The miller, therefore, adds chemicals to the flour which bleach and mature it in a couple of days. For many years, the bleaching and maturing nitrogen trichloride agent, agene, was used. In 1946, agene-treated flour was fed to dogs in a medical experiment and produced a form of hysteria in them. The agene agent was banned, and flour is still legally bleached but with chlorine, chlorine dioxide, and other chemicals. The longterm effect of chlorinated fats in the flour has not been examined, but we do know that nitrogen trichloride reacts with an amino acid, methionine, to form methionine sulphoximine, which causes epileptic-like seizures. Chlorine will do the same. Bleaching destroys both carotene (the precursor of vitamin A) and vitamin E, and it leaves chlorinated residues of amino acids and fats. Other chemicals, for example, potassium bromate, are "improving" or "maturing" agents that have no bleaching effect.

In 1820, the French physiologist, F. Magendie, found that coarse dark bread kept dogs in good health, while feeding them bread made from white flour saw the dogs die within two months. The *Lancet*, March 11, 1826, reported, "A dog fed on fine white bread and water, both at discretion, does not live beyond the fiftieth day. A dog fed on the coarse bread of the military, lives and keeps his health." Since then, there has been a vigorous debate between the supporters of whole wheat bread and the supporters of white bread.

As a cereal chemist, one of us, (A.H.), was involved for several years on the side of the white bread group. I was a typical food technologist and assumed that in any balanced diet, white bread was as nutritious as whole wheat bread, especially if it was enriched with thiamine, riboflavin, niacinamide, and iron. Since 90 percent of the public seemed to prefer white bread, it seemed appropriate to provide them with what they wanted. Over the past forty years, white bread has remained the staple for the majority of the population. A small proportion, perhaps 15 percent, were nutritionally aware and consumed only whole grain breads. Only in Great Britain, during the last war, did white bread give way to a darker product, but this was a logistical decision, not a nutritional one. By milling darker flour, Britain could import less wheat and could use its ships instead to haul munitions. Sugar was rationed. Coincidentally, there was a marked improvement in the overall health of the people which terminated after the war when once more Britons had access to all the sugar and white flour they had a taste for.

The Public Is Fooled by Food Processors

Processing can be divided into three phases: (a) refining of grains and animal products to obtain proteins, fats, and starches; (b) treatment of the refined product by chemical procedures that change their molecular structure; and (c) fabrication into the final products. At each stage, chemical additives are used, each carrying its quota of trace impurities, and natural nutrients are lost.

The whole science of food processing is predicated on fooling the public into thinking it is getting nutritional value when it is not. The result is that the degradation of real food into fake food probably is bringing on early aging and senility.

Most of the degradation previously occurred in fats and starches but proteins are now being destroyed in the same way. The public is becoming aware that sugars and processed starches are dangerous but so far have not been alerted to the equally dangerous protein extenders. The word "protein" or "high-protein food" still carries a connotation of a high quality, nutritious food, especially for those interested in hypoglycemia and for vegetarians who want only plant proteins.

Soybeans contain protein and are good high-protein foods, but they taste unpleasant—like soybeans. Soybean protein is converted into textured vegetable protein (T.V.P.), and designed to look and taste like chicken, ham, steak or turkey. This is how it is done: the protein is removed from ground soybean with petroleum solvent, alcohol and hydrochloric acid. The refined protein is dissolved in alkali which is then precipitated into an acid bath as filaments. These filament threads are soaked in artificial binders, flavor and colors. The cemented fibers are mixed with fat and a few minerals and vitamins to simulate the natural meats, but they are synthetics. Synthetic meats have not been shown to be safe over longterm use. Dr. George M. Buggs, a nutritionist at the University of California, Berkeley, labels them "a nutritional step backwards." These food artifacts are advertised in such a way as to lead the unwary to believe they are as nutritious as the meat they simulate, when in truth they will probably be proven toxic over the long haul.

In 1940, about 20 percent of our food was processed; today it is closer to 80 percent. This means that most people depend heavily on food prepared for them by industry. The rapid development of convenience foods, and the decreased status awarded homemakers have played major roles.

Convenience foods are attractively packaged, can be stored for a long time, require little work and no culinary skill, and are palatable. The commercial advertising on radio, television, in newspapers and magazines emphasize the wisdom in selecting Brand "A" over any other food. The homemaker is extolled because she knew enough to open up a can of Brand "A" food, not because of her skill in selecting a food which will nourish and keep her family healthy.

Processed food includes everything derived from food

but which has been ripped out of food. It is treated and recombined into what appears to be food. Actually it is invariably only a fraction as nutritious (in terms of supporting life) as the original food.

As we implied, white flour is made from the least nutritious portion of the wheat kernel lacking vitamins and minerals.

Sugar is the least nutritious fraction of the sugar beet or cane. The word *nutritious* used here is inappropriate. It is more correct to say that sugar is the most toxic, poisonous, fraction of these plants. It is a fraction which provides calories only in the absence of all the essential components of food.

Processed food also contains chemicals which are added to improve certain properties such as color, flavor, and resistance against deterioration. The chemicals add nothing to the nutritional quality and are toxic for many people. There is no requirement that foods adulterated with these chemicals must be safe as would be the case if the same chemical were to be introduced into medicine as a drug. Theoretically, tranquilizers could be introduced into our food, if they were shown to prevent oxidation or rancidity. And they might have these properties, indeed, since they are large molecules which could remove metallic ions from enzymes and so inactivate them. These enzymes are partially responsible for oxidation of a food on its standing. There is no requirement that processed food must be as nutritious as the food from which it has been made. We have adapted to food during evolution, not to the food artifact created from processing techniques.

The Derivation of Food Artifacts by the Food Processing Industry

Over hundreds of milennia, we have adapted to natural food—it is food that is alive such as seeds and vegetables, or food that recently has been alive, like meat and fish.

There has been little deterioration from the time the food was harvested and consumed. Natural nutrition has been the pattern followed by hunting peoples, even among those who are still hunters, such as the primitive Kung people.

With the development of agriculture and cities, it became necessary to feed a population far from where the food was gathered. The supply had to be stored for long periods of time. With vegetables, this did not alter their nutritional quality much until modern chemistry created food technology. Briefly, this is an elaborate modern system for converting food into food artifact. We will present the evidence that this technological change in what we eat is to a large measure responsible for our current health crises and for a major increase in senility. But before we can do so, we will outline ways of thinking about food and food artifacts.

Modern food technology developed from chemistry and brought into existence a whole new industry of food processing. Chemists of the nineteenth century discovered that if they subjected food to certain chemical procedures, specific fractions of the food were isolated. Any chemist following the same procedure could isolate the same kind of material. The substances were purified and were found to have particular characteristic properties.

One of these substances was called *protein*, consisting of long chain molecules made up by a series of small molecules called *amino acids*. Proteins contain nitrogen.

Another type of material was oily and dissolved in fat solvents more than in water. They did not contain nitrogen, and were either short or long chain hydrocarbons. They are the lipids or fats.

The third major material was carbohydrate, comprising starch cellulose and sugars.

Once these substances were isolated and their properties recognized, chemists and later nutritionists began to think of foods as so much protein, fat and carbohydrate. But in nature, these substances do not exist in pure form, nor do they have the properties characteristic of food. In food, we have a very complex mixture of protein, fat, and carbohydrate molecules. These fractions are food artifacts because they are the products of chemical ingenuity. If these methods had not been discovered, we would know nothing of protein, fat and carbohydrates and have no food processing industry.

When we swallow food, it is ground, mixed with enzymes, and digested. During digestion, the protein, fat and carbohydrates are released more or less at the same time, gradually and slowly. The amino acids, fats and sugars, are released slowly and absorbed slowly. Large amounts are not dumped into the blood and do not stress the liver and other digestive organs but are regulated in their uptake.

Artifacts are not digested in the same way as are whole foods. Protein artifacts have been altered by chemical processing as have fat artifacts, and the digestion of them is different. Starches and sugars derived from processing are digested too quickly, dumping large quantities of sugar into the blood. Such dumping plays havoc with the pancreas, liver, and the entire digestive apparatus.

Food artifacts can be reconstituted into artifact concoctions which have no similarity to food, and which have not been proven to be nutritious. There are no studies that show corn flakes to be as nutritious as the original corn nor are there studies that show white flour to be as nutritious as whole wheat flour. On the contrary, there are a large number of studies which prove that artifacts and their combinations are much less nutritious than the food from which they have been extracted.

Food also contains vitamins, minerals, enzymes, and other molecules which are essential for health. It is dangerous and naive to assume that every essential nutrient had already been identified. Separate nutrients also are artifacts. In food, vitamins and minerals are bound to, or are component parts of, the other food components. They, too, are realized slowly by the body through its digestive system. These extra nutrients are absorbed slowly along with the other food derivatives with no rapid increases in concentration in blood, and less loss in urine due to surpassing the renal threshold.

Food seldom contains such a large quantity of any one food artifact that its consumption is dangerous. Thus, it is possible to live on a diet of almost pure meats. This contains protein and fat. But living on protein alone, free of fat, can be very dangerous. The food processors have now given us textured protein made from vegetable sources to eat; too much of this material will be harmful.

The most dangerous artifacts produced by processing are the carbohydrates, especially the sugars. They actually cause disability and bring on early death.

We must stop thinking of food as protein, fat or carbohydrates. It is better to think of protein-rich, fat-rich or carbohydrate-rich *whole* food. We will continue to discuss protein, fats and carbohydrates in this book, because of convenience; we must not forget, however, that these are artifacts—not foods—merely capital-producers for the food processing industry.

Food processing industrialists have been sensitive to the charge that they produce unhealthy foods. Fortunately for them, they have been able to obtain cover by government sponsored food guides or rules. Of these, the most pernicious rule is the myth of the balanced diet. It is true that all the nutrients must be provided and that a diet balanced by choosing items from various types of foods such as vegetables, nuts, seeds, fruit, and meat will be adequate for most people. But this rule, formulated several decades ago, is no longer adequate when so much of our daily intake consists of junk.

A balanced diet consists of a balance of foods. You can't balance inadequate food artifacts as food and have a nutritious diet. The extreme to which this term is used is represented by those ads which claim that an ounce of cereal with four ounces of milk provides a balanced meal.

They do not claim that this combination is any more nutritious than four ounces of milk alone; to illustrate it in another way, one can claim that sawdust combined with milk is an equally nutritious food. Obviously, this kind of advertising is misleading. The addition of some food artifact, such as junk cereal, can only decrease the nutritional quality of any food with which it is mixed.

It is also said by the processors in defense of junk food, that one does not live on that alone. No one eats only sugar, or white bread or sugared drinks. But what is not said is that the drift toward junk food of twenty years ago has become a stampede. So much of our daily intake is junk and, unfortunately, there is not enough food consumed to make up for the nutritional inadequacies of the junk.

It is now possible to have entirely artifact-filled meals such as Egg Beaters, sausage, artificial tomato catsup, white bread, jam, and Tang for breakfast; artificial hamburgers, potato chips, apple pie, and ice cream and coffee with sugar for lunch; canned soup, canned peas and carrots, steak, canned pears, wine, and tea with sugar for dinner. The only real food in this total litany is the steak which may be over-cooked and covered with the artificial flavor enhancers containing glutamate, too much salt and other spices. Over 90 percent of the full listing furnished here is utter junk. Where is our concept of eating the balanced diet then, when many people eat this way?

Today, one-third of all meals eaten in Canada and the United States are away from home in restaurants, institutions, airplanes, ships and elsewhere. Soon it will be 50 percent of the public depending on out-of-home dining to assuage hunger. There are not many restaurants that provide real food; most rely heavily on processed convenience items which need only to be heated to get them out of the kitchen to the customer fast.

The result? We are a nation suffering from subtle, chronic malnutrition, not from lack of quantity taken into our bodies but from an absence of quality in the nutrition we attempt. Senility has to be one of the degenerative processes that affect our nerves and arteries from this sort of wrong practice. We affront nature by thinking our food technologists can duplicate her handiwork. The food processors have duped us with their promises of time savings, less work in food preparation, easy recipes, better taste, attractive dishes, varying menus, vitamin fortification and the other advertising lies. What we actually buy when we take their products into our homes are premature aging, senility, heart trouble and other forms of disability—the diseases of degeneration. These diseases of malnutrition amidst affluence and abundance is the topic of our next chapter.

References for Chapter Four

1. Nutrition experts urge study of elderly's needs. *The New York Times*, June 7, 1978.

2. Stieglitz, E.J. *Geriatric Medicine*, 2nd. Ed. Philadelphia: W.B. Saunders, 1949.

3. Stieglitz, E.J. Nutrition problems of geriatric medicine. *Journal of the American Medical Association* 142: 1070-1077, 1950.

4. Droller, H. and Dossett, J.A. *Geriatrics* 14:367, 1959.

5. Kral, V.A. Senescence and forgetfulness: benign and malignant. *Canadian Medical Assocation Journal* 86:257-260, 1962.

5

DEGENERATIVE DISEASES CAUSED BY CONSUMING FOOD ARTIFACTS

Although people insist on examining all the diets of the world looking for one component, such as cholesterol, to blame as a cause of heart disease, they would be doing better to look for the absence of one component, such as vitamin E. Just as it is dangerous to worry only about cholesterol, it is dangerous to worry only about vitamin E. Total nutrition—Supernutrition—is the main concern. Without it, we are predisposed to premature heart disease.
—Richard A. Passwater, Ph.D., *Supernutrition*, 1975

A Minor Curb on "Junk Food" in Schools Proposed

ON JULY 6, 1979, Carol Tucker Foreman, a former head of the Consumer Federation of America and now the Assistant Secretary of the U.S. Department of Agriculture, officially proposed a ban on "junk food" covering such items as sodas, chewing gum, frozen desserts and some candies in the public schools. The USDA had spent almost two years working to define "junk food" and propose the new rule. About 98 percent of the nation's public schools serving federally subsidized lunches would be affected by the junk food ban beginning January 1, 1980.

At first appearance, it looks as if a victory has been gained by exponents of orthomolecular nutrition and the coauthors of this book. School children who want to buy non-nutritional snacks and soft drinks from school vending machines or cafeterias would have to wait until the day's last lunch is served under this rule. More than 25.7 million American children would be forced to comply and, theoretically, be saved from early aging and eventual senility because of better nutrition in their formative years. Vending machine operators might be encouraged to offer fruits, vegetables, fruit juices and nuts instead of "foods of minimum nutritional value," as the Department of Agriculture labels the junk.[1]

In truth, the victory is hollow indeed, for the proposal still would permit most foods with minimal nutritional value. Junk with less than 5 percent of the recommended daily allowance (RDA) of any one of eight basic nutrients won't be acceptable. But the full schedule of RDAs are already inadequate, as we've pointed out in prior chapters. Would you permit just 5 percent now of such a low standard?

The proposed rules define junk foods as a 100-calorie portion containing 5 percent of the RDA of vitamin A, vitamin C, protein, vitamin B-3, vitamin B-1, vitamin B-2, calcium or iron. No rules were set down as to maximum salt, sugar or fat content. Jody Levin-Epstein, an assistant to Mrs. Foreman, said:

> If a candy bar has only one nut in it, we feel it is above our minimum nutrient standards. We hope schools will build on the spirit of this ruling and go even further with it, as many states and cities already have.

Michael F. Jacobson, Ph.D., Director of the Center for Science in the Public Interest, points out that much of the candy now being sold would continue to be sold because it meets the 5 percent minimum. He said the government should have required a maximum sugar content as well. "I think it's almost a total cave-in to the snack food industry," declared Dr. Jacobson. "It just doesn't rectify the situation."

He called the new USDA rule "a farce, a cruel joke" and

said it would allow the sale in schools of most candies and even "sugar-coated grease balls."[2]

Consumer activist Ralph Nader said he agreed with Jacobson's critical assessment of the rule and told reporters: "I don't know how Carol Foreman allowed this one to go through." Nader, members of the Consumer Federation of America, the Parent Teacher Association and others speculate that the snack food industry will just slightly increase the nutritional content of their products to meet the 5 percent figure.

What has happened? The Department of Agriculture has bowed to the snack food industry lobby in Washington. It has compromised itself and accepted an inadequate proposal to relieve itself of pressure. David Stratman, director of government relations for the PTA, confirmed this. In 1978, he said, the PTA endorsed a stronger rule against the sale of junk foods in schools, but that the government later withdrew it because of pressure from the snack food industry.

Agriculture Department spokesman Jim Webster conceded that the rule is a compromise that was reached after the department's previous proposal was criticized by the snack food industry.

In effect, the government has conceded that it can't reduce the incidence of food artifact usage. Food will continue to be divided into separate proteins, fats and carbohydrates fostering conditions whereby hardening of the arteries and other degenerative diseases will perpetuate among our young. All junk foods should be banished or the restrictions to them extended for the entire school day, but as of now, this is not the case.

The Food Artifacts That Perpetuate Degenerative Diseases

Chapter Four describes how food artifacts are derived by food processors who have built a highly lucrative industry through sophisticated technology. They split our components from whole foods and sell them separately in the form of protein, fat and carbohydrate products. Today, that industry is a trillion dollar operation in Western industrialized countries. So much money and power are not easily turned aside by a mere government edict.

To better understand how food artifacts perpetuate degenerative diseases in our population, we will discuss the separate components—the food artifacts—extracted from whole food. Eating singular components, that is, just protein or fat or carbohydrate, is a practice quite hazardous to your health. We will explain why.

Protein artifacts in the form of reconstituted concoctions were also discussed in the last chapter. Proteins, composed of amino acids, are essential for health. Of the twenty required, eight cannot be made in the body and are considered the essential amino acids. Foods rich in protein are judged to be of high or low quality, depending upon the amount of essential amino acid present. A high quality protein-rich food will support growth and life better than a low quality protein.

The diet must contain enough protein to maintain repair and growth, something that varies for different individuals. It is best to consume a slight protein surplus to ensure enough at all times, especially when the body is under severe stress. Generally, too little is much more dangerous than too much. For your own body, you must make a decision as to what is the optimal amount.

Whenever possible, obtain your protein from a whole food and not from protein artifacts. Protein artifacts should be used only as a concentrated source of essential amino acids. This is one way of improving the quality of protein-rich food.

The Fat Artifacts

Fats are extracted from, or pressed from, foods with high fat content to provide a more concentrated form of energy. One gram of fat artifact provides nine calories of energy as compared to four calories per gram of protein or carbohydrate. Fats give the main reservoir of energy in animals, which is an advantage since carbohydrates in bulk are bulky and rigid. In contrast, fats at body temperature are fluid and yield to movement. If we were to store our excess calories as carbohydrate, we would be more obese and quite stiff—more like a tree or a potato than like an animal. Plants store energy primarily as carbohydrates and also to a lesser degree as fat.

Fats are composed of fatty acids of various lengths and with different degrees of saturation. A fat which has no double bonds in it tends to be rigid, like wax, from being fully hydrogenated. Fats which contain double bonds are more fluid and contain less hydrogen. An unsaturated fat can be saturated by adding hydrogen, which is how liquid fats or oils are converted into some solid fats like margarine. Enough hydrogen is added to create the same melting or liquification point of butter. A variety of fatty acids are required for health ranging from short chain acids like butyric acid, to very long chain acids. The long fatty acids must be in the diet: they are considered essential fatty acids.

All natural fats are "cis" molecules. That means there is a constant three dimensional relationship of the atoms to each other. The enzymes in the body are designed to metabolize these molecules. There is another way the atoms can be put together called "trans," but no natural enzymes exist for these. When liquid fats are hydrogenated, up to 50 percent of the "cis" molecules are converted into "trans" molecules. When you consume margarine, up to one-half is not digestible in the body and gets excreted as waste.

Fats are required because they are essential components of our body; they provide a low bulk, energy-rich source; many processes including absorption of vitamins soluble in fat require the presence of fat. Too little fat may cause a variety of undesirable reactions, and too much fat will cause obesity.

Usually a person can depend upon his palate to tell how much fat is needed. Foods too low in fat tend to be less appetizing, and foods too rich in fat too greasy. The palate is perverted, however, if fats are blended with sugars as in ice cream. Then, huge quantities of fat may be consumed in ice cream and other concoctions. The optimum amount of fat varies from individual to individual. Obese and overweight individuals should eliminate all sugars and then cut back, but not eliminate, fats as well as protein.

There are other substances which have fat properties such as cholesterol, lecithin and a few others. The idea that too much cholesterol in the diet causes coronary disease is widespread among physicians. This belief has led to the use of low fat diets, which in itself would cause no harm, but a low fat diet in most cases leads to an increase in the consumption of carbohydrate artifacts, especially the sugars. If fats were restricted and sugars eliminated, we could not quarrel with such a diet, but by focusing almost entirely on fats (cholesterol), the vital role of sugars in causing coronary disease has been overlooked. This may explain why exclusively low fat diets have been relatively ineffective in lowering the incidence of coronary disease.

The relationship between fats in the food and coronary disease has been examined seriously by Richard A. Passwater, Ph.D., who has concluded that there is no correlation between fat content of food and cholesterol and triglyceride levels in the blood. Populations who consume a lot of foods rich in fats may be free of coronary disease, and populations on low fat diets may have as much coronary disease as we do in North America.

A modern program recommended for decreasing the incidence or the possibility of developing coronary disease consists of four changes in one's pattern of living. These are: (1) to relax; (2) to eliminate smoking; (3) to exercise; and (4) to reduce consumption of fat artifacts. All four recommendations are excellent, and we urge every individual to follow them.

The residents of St. Helena, either as a result of fate or of geography, observe all four points. They tend to be relaxed compared to other populations. By tradition, they do not smoke very heavily. They are not heavy consumers of fat, and because the island is hilly and there are few vehicles, they get a lot of exercise getting from place to place. One would expect that they would have a low incidence of coronary disease. When Shine, in his book, *Serendipity on St. Helena*,[3] examined the population, he found that the incidence of coronary disease was as high as in England. An examination of the data on consumption of foods showed that the St. Helenans' consumption of sugar was similar to that in England, about 120 pounds per year per person. The relationship between coronary disease and sugar will be examined in the next section. Under this section on fats, we have included this information to demonstrate that fats were not implicated as a major factor in causing coronary disease on St. Helena. If these fat artifacts (like butter and oil) were not heavily implicated, then it is obvious fat-rich foods might have even less connection. These foods do possess a major defect; they are rich in calories and may lead to obesity in those unable to control their food intake.

While it is true that people with high blood cholesterol and/or high blood triglycerides are more apt to suffer from coronary disease, it does not follow that one causes the other. Both are the result of other biochemical problems, probably symptoms of the Saccharine Disease described by T.L. Cleave, M.R.C.P., former Surgeon-Captain in the Royal Navy. When blood fats are elevated, the individual is warned that a change in life style, with perhaps the use of specific treatment, is imperative.

Hardening of the arteries is a prominent factor leading to senility. If the hardening occurs in the heart arteries, the heart can't efficiently pump blood through the body, and the brain is especially sensitive to a decreased blood flow. If this reduced flow continues for a long time, there will be deterioration in the brain. A steady loss of brain neurons must lead to organic deterioration of the brain ending in senility.

Arteriosclerosis in the vessels of the brain will have the same effect as reduction of blood flow everywhere else. There will be a decreased activity in all parts. The human body must be used. If any function is allowed to atrophy, it will have some effect upon the rest of the body, including the brain.

Cholesterol and Hardening of the Arteries

We have referred to the idea that cholesterol is a cause of arteriosclerosis. One of us, (A.H.), was very sympathetic to this idea over twenty years ago. In 1954, I developed the conviction that vitamin B-3 was therapeutic for acute or early schizophrenic patients. In our research group in Saskatchewan, we had completed the first double blind experiment ever recorded in psychiatric literature, the testing of nucleotides only on acute and chronic schizophrenics. In a second study, testing was done comparing nicotinic acid and nicotinamide against placebo. The three experimental treatments were incorporated into the standard program then current—psychotherapy and electroconvulsive therapy (ECT). One year after the last patient had been treated, the state of all the patients was examined and recorded. On breaking the treatment code, we found that the addition of vitamin B-3 doubled the one-year recovery rate from the usual 35 percent rate expected as a natural recovery rate, to an unusual 70 percent recovery.

There were no tranquilizers then. Even today, the improvement rate with tranquilizers is not much better than the natural untreated rate. A survey of schizophrenics treated in Massachusetts between 1945 and 1949, when there were no tranquilizers, and 1965 to 1969, when they were the only standard treatment, revealed no difference in outcome. If anything, the early group was better off.

Apparently, tranquilizers as the main treatment not only did not help them recover, but made the patients more dependent on welfare and other agencies.

In 1954, Professor Rudl Altschul, Chairman, Department of Anatomy, of the University of Saskatchewan, approached me with his discovery that ultraviolet light lowered cholesterol levels in rabbits and in patients. He wanted to enlarge his series of human subjects, but could not find any physicians who would cooperate with him. In my role as Director of Psychiatric Research, Professor Altschul knew I had access to several thousand patients. Ultraviolet irradiation (like sunlight) as he proposed to use it seemed not to be harmful and might, in fact, be beneficial because very few of my patients had much opportunity to be in the sun. I felt that the increased attention focused on the patients because of the research would be psychologically helpful to them. Dr. H. Osmond, Medical Superintendent of the mental hospital at Weyburn, Saskatchewan, agreed with me.

A few weeks later, I met Altschul at the railroad station and we drove to Weyburn, seventy-two miles away. On the way there and back, we discussed our research interests. Altschul had been a neuro-psychiatrist in Prague when he was forced to leave Europe in 1939. He was invited to join the Department of Anatomy, University of Saskatchewan, as an instructor and later became chairman of the department. He could not practice medicine as the College of Physicians and Surgeons insisted he intern for one year before they would allow him to practice. Altschul refused to give up his work for the year and switched his interests instead. He became very involved in research into arteriosclerosis, finally becoming an international authority.

The professor believed that the main factor in the development of hardening of the arteries was a pathological change in the intima, the thin layer of cells which made up the inner lining of each blood vessel, by losing its ability to repair itself. He was also interested in cholesterol levels since it had been shown that high blood cholesterol levels were associated with increased deposition of arteriosclerotic plaques.

Rabbits normally do not develop hardening of the arteries, probably because of their high consumption of high fiber food. When rabbits are fed rations very rich in cholesterol such as eggs, they still do not become ill. If however, the egg yolk is prepared in a cake and baked, this food then elevates cholesterol levels quickly. The heating process converts a healthy food into a substance which is pathological for rabbits. Having rabbits available with high cholesterol levels, it was possible to try various procedures such as ultraviolet irradiation to lower cholesterol levels. As Prof. Altschul continued to discuss these ideas, I became more and more interested in the idea that the intima had lost its ability to heal itself as well.

For many months, I had been annoyed by bleeding gums. Many visits to my dentist and large doses of ascorbic acid did not help. The problem was that I had some malocclusion—some of my teeth did not meet head-on. As a result, when I chewed there was increased pressure and strain between the tooth and socket. I had concluded that my tissues were less able to repair themselves and were beginning to break down and that there was no treatment except eventually to extract my teeth. About this time, I had started to take nicotinic acid, 1 gram, three times per day. I wanted to see what the effect would be on me, both unpleasant (side effects) and beneficial. About two weeks later, I was astonished when my toothbrush was no longer red with blood when I brushed. My gums had become normal, something my dentist confirmed had happened at the next visit. This was such a surprising event I could not forget it.

I tried to reason why the vitamin had been so helpful and ruled out any placebo effect. I had not expected any improvement whatever; had not taken it for any therapeutic reason as I felt well, and no one has yet shown that any placebo has cured severe swelling and inflammation of the gums. I eventually hypothesized that the vitamin restored the ability of my tissues, in which my teeth were embedded, to repair themselves.

When Altschul spoke about repair of the intima, I immediately brought up my personal experience with the niacin. It occurred to me that niacin might also restore the ability of the intima to repair itself and thus might prevent or reverse the damage caused by arteriosclerosis. Altschul asked where he could get some, and I promised to send him a pound of pure crystalline niacin. This I did and then no longer thought about it.

Several months later, I received a phone call from Prof. Rudl Altschul. He was very excited, shouting at me, "It works, it works!" I did not know what he was talking about until he told me he had given niacin to his rabbits who suffered from chronic high blood cholesterol because they were fed cooked egg yolk. Their cholesterol levels promptly became normal.

He asked how he might find patients with high blood cholesterol. I offered to do the study at General Hospital, Regina, where I had the research program for the province. The next day, I approached the hospital pathologist and outlined my problem to him. Could he help locate a number of patients? He agreed to do so. Within a few days, Dr. J. Stephen had located about seventy patients, all in the hospital.

After their cholesterol levels were measured, they were given niacin, 3 grams per day, for two days. Then their cholesterol levels were remeasured. This very quick study and brief series showed that niacin lowered cholesterol in people as well as in rabbits. The higher the pretreatment levels were, the greater was the cholesterol decrease. We published our results in 1955 in a paper by Altschul, Hoffer and Stephen.[4]

Even then, the resistance against vitamins was so great that our findings were rejected, with the first public comment appearing in an abstract of our paper in *Nutrition Reviews*. The author was so convinced that niacin could not lower cholesterol (even though he had never tested it) that he incorrectly read our basic table. By misreading this table, he was able to prove (he thought) that there was no decrease in cholesterol whatever. A few months later, *Nutrition Reviews* published my letter that pointed out this blatant error.

Since that early study, over 1200 papers have been published confirming our research work. The hypocholesterolemic property of megadoses of niacin is the only one recognized by the FDA, which illustrates that major discoveries often arise from very inexpensive research. Niacin was the first substance ever shown to lower cholesterol levels and triglyceride levels, but because it is an orphan drug, it has not been widely promoted.

In 1955, I recommended to the Department of Public Health, Government of Saskatchewan, that they take out a patent on niacin's hypocholesterol action. We had one year following the publication of our paper in which to file a patent application, but the Department refused to act. Had they followed my advice, niacin would have been patented. It would have been licensed to a drug company —acquired parents—a company interested in its promotion.

Another nonphysiological compound, Atromid, also lowers cholesterol. It is widely known and used since its discovery. Its parents—large drug companies—have continually reminded physicians of its effectiveness by means of colorful, skillfully drawn ads.

We therefore have a situation where a nonphysiological drug, Atromid, which lowers cholesterol and has no other beneficial effect is used widely, while a natural nutrient, niacin, which has a large number of beneficial properties including the ability to lower blood fat levels, is widely ignored.

Had the Government of Saskatchewan shown any imagination, it would have established niacin long before Atromid came on the scene, and would have a continuing source of revenue. The Government may have been motivated by its desire not to profit from any medical discovery, but I think this unlikely. The bureaucrats simply did not have enough vision to foresee what could have happened. They were not aware that no treatment or drug will be sold unless there is money in it for a drug company. No company can distribute and advertise a product unless they can expect to recapture their costs and make a profit. This has been recognized by the law regulating distribution of drugs in Canada and the United States. There is no provision in law for an individual physician to distribute any drug. It was assumed by law that only drug companies would do so.

Since our early work, I have retained my interest in cholesterol metabolism and how it is altered by the vitamin, niacin. However, it has become clear that other vitamins and other nutritional factors play major roles as well.

Elevated cholesterol levels indicate there is something wrong with the metabolism of the body. Just lowering cholesterol by interfering with its synthesis as is done by some drugs is not good enough, if the basic disease remains unchecked. I fully expect that patients whose hypercholesterolemia is controlled by drugs such as Atromid will continue to suffer from the basic disease, of which their elevated cholesterol is merely a symptom. In fact, a very large study in the U.S.A. showed that just lowering cholesterol with Atromid or with niacin did not halt the progress of arteriosclerosis and coronary death. Long-term use of Atromid will keep cholesterol levels down, but has no other beneficial effect, nor is there much evidence it prevents coronary disease.

A clinical study recently completed in England, if confirmed, will be the end of Atromid's use. In this study, it was found that patients given Atromid to reduce cholesterol levels had a much higher death rate than a control group. There was also a higher incidence of gall bladder disease requiring surgery, and of those operated on, a much higher proportion died. This leaves us with only one safe broad spectrum hypolipidemic agent—niacin.

Niacin will keep cholesterol levels down, but it has so many other beneficial effects that its use is warranted on a routine basis. As a nutrient, it is bound in the long run to be much safer than Atromid. Atromid is a compound not normally found in the body which therefore has no way of dealing with it. As with most drugs, it acts because of some toxic effect on some enzymes in the body. This is not the case for the vitamins. They are not toxic even though a large quantitiy of a vitamin might interfere with some reactions because of the large number of molecules present. A toxic drug may be compared to having a kidnapper in the house who prevents one from getting food from the table. Starvation is the result. Having too much vitamin around is like having so many friends in the house that it is almost impossible to get to the table. In both cases, the person is hungry. But I would rather be hungry surrounded by friends (friendly molecules) than by enemies (toxic molecules).

The Absent Relationship Between Senility and Cholesterol

Because it is widely believed that food cholesterol and arteriosclerosis are related, it is important to present the existing evidence that food cholesterol and arteriosclerosis are not related—the full cholesterol controversy. This, therefore, means that there is little relationship between senility and food cholesterol.

Cholesterol is another artifact extracted from food or other material by using fat solvents. In nature, cholesterol does not exist in a pure form but is a component of tissues of the body. It composes a major proportion of the dry weight of the brain and is used by the body to make bile salts, hormones, and vitamin D-3. Around 1.5 to 2 grams is made each day by the average person. No one eats pure cholesterol, but we do eat foods containing cholesterol such as dairy products, eggs and organ meats. Nonetheless, food provides only a small proportion of our daily cholesterol requirement; the rest is made in the body. If more is consumed, less need be made. For this reason, healthy people who eat just whole food have little to fear.

Cholesterol is made from carbohydrates and an excessive intake of sugar and/or of fat can increase cholesterol levels. However, sugar and fat are food artifacts which should not be part of any person's food intake.

It is generally believed that there is a wide range of normal human cholesterol levels, usually between 150 and 250 mg per 100 ml of blood. Some laboratories accept even higher levels as normal, a practice we believe to be a serious error. There are many people around with these higher levels who are not considered to be ill, and what is common is assumed to be normal. Using this line of reasoning, if a community of people were found with one blind eye, this would be construed to be normal. High cholesterol levels indicate there is something seriously wrong with the metabolism, and it must be corrected. When it is corrected, the cholesterol levels will return to normal. If patients with 300 mg of cholesterol per 100 ml of blood are assured there is nothing wrong, they will not be motivated to do something about their imbalanced nutrition.

We believe that the normal cholesterol range is 150 to 200 mg percent, and that a desirable optimum is around 160 mg percent. Many years ago, I studied the effect of niacin on the cholesterol levels of a large number of patients. I found that the amount of change depended upon the original levels. In other words, the more abnormal the problem was as measured by cholesterol levels, the more effective was the corrective response. If cholesterol levels were less than 165 mg percent, they were elevated to that level. Several patients with levels below 120 mg were at 150, or better, while taking niacin. Cholesterol levels over 165 were decreased, with the greatest decrease coming from very high levels. I had then concluded that it was more accurate to consider niacin a normalizer of cholesterol levels rather than a hypocholesterolemic agent. Practically, it made no difference, since the vast majority of patients have too much, not too little blood cholesterol; but the great theoretical significance of this observation has been ignored. Instead of searching for the mechanism by which niacin lowers cholesterol, scientists should have been looking for those aspects of metabolism normalized by niacin.

The idea that food rich in cholesterol causes hardening of the arteries with consequent coronary disease has paved the way for the food processing industries to provide special foods with little cholesterol. A second idea that polyunsaturated fats will lower cholesterol levels has created food artifacts high in these fats. Both these approaches, which seemed sound many years ago, have turned out to be incorrect.

The food processing industry is more sensitive to consumer pressure than it is to scientific discovery. So far, the consumers who are aware that foods are not villains, although food artifacts are, have not created enough pressure on food processors to moderate their advertising message.

Two basic but incorrect propositions should be examined: Do foods rich in cholesterol cause arteriosclerosis and coronary disease? Do unsaturated fats have any beneficial value in preventing heart and vascular disease?

The first proposition is true if the following statements are true:

1. Cholesterol-rich foods increase blood fats to abnormally high levels.
2. Abnormally elevated cholesterol levels is a cause of arteriosclerosis.

Extensive research has shown that each statement is mostly wrong. There are a large number of people and groups of people who eat a lot of cholesterol-rich foods with normal or low blood cholesterol levels. Conversely, there are many people and groups of people who eat foods low in cholesterol who have high blood cholesterol levels. The correlation between cholesterol content of food and cholesterol levels in the blood is so slight that very large series of patients must be studied in order to find a statistically significant relationship. Even with a correlation coefficient of 0.5 which would be extremely high, cholesterol-rich foods would account for only 25 percent of the variance, and other factors would be three times as important. With a correlation of 0.4 which is more likely, the variance drops to 16 percent, leaving 84 percent of the factors to be accounted for by other factors.

The correlation between blood cholesterol levels and the coronary occlusions is somewhat closer. This is not surprising since the basic metabolic fault which causes both elevated cholesterol levels and coronary disease would ensure such a relationship. In the same way, the two front wheels of a wagon are correlated even if the propulsive power does not come from either one. A correlation does not prove cause and effect, while a lack of correlation disproves it. The correlation between triglycerides and coronary disease is closer still, indicating that triglyceride levels may be a better indicator of the basic metabolic fault which leads to arteriosclerosis.

Since there is such a low relationship, there seems little point in trying to lower cholesterol levels without doing something about the basic metabolic fault. To give hypocholesterolemic substances while ignoring those factors which are responsible, seems inappropriate. In combination with proper nutrition and essential nutrient supplements, these hypocholesterolemic compounds are valuable.

There is some evidence that polyunsaturated fats will lower cholesterol levels. Since these are artifacts, however, all the evidence of the harmful effects of artifacts applies as well. There is no evidence that foods rich in these vegetable fats have any significant effect. Polyunsaturated fats contain less hydrogen and are liquid at room temperature. Thus, safflower oil or corn oil are more unsaturated than the fat in milk, which we know better as *butter*. The American Heart Association has reported there is no conclusive proof that these fats prevent heart disease. They should have made their statement stronger by stating there is a good deal of evidence; there is such a slight relationship that it is heavily outweighed by the possible toxicity of polyunsaturated fats.

Diets rich in polyunsaturates have been shown to deplete vitamin E from the body. These fats possess highly reactive double bonds which have an affinity for other atoms. In saturated fats, these reactive bonds disappear. The unsaturated fats are easily oxidized within the body and outside the body. In the body, they produce exceedingly reactive free radicals which increase cross linkages (thereby creating blockages). Vitamin E destroys these free radicals. There is an increased demand for vitamin E and much more is required. The increased production of free radicals is one of the factors inducing premature aging and senility. When heated, these polyunsaturates form toxic polymers that are highly oxidized. Fats or fat-rich foods fried too much become much more toxic. Animals fed too much polyunsaturated fats have lost their hair, been stunted, and died earlier. These fats have also been linked with circulatory sludging. Finally, data has been accumulated to suggest that these fats increase the possibility of cancer and arteriosclerosis, premature aging and reduced life span.

All the evidence we have referred to reinforces our conclusion that no one need fear whole food, whether it is rich in fat, protein or carbohydrate. What is to be feared and avoided are the food artifacts whether they are rich in protein, carbohydrates or fats. Since there is a relationship of cholesterol to circulatory disease, and no connection to food, then it is obvious that there will be even less to cerebral vascular disorders and to senility. There are many factors causing senility which we should worry about and correct. The consumption of cholesterol-rich food is not among the main ones.

In concluding this section on the cholesterol artifact we have to point out that Dr. Mark D. Altschule rejects the idea that cholesterol causes atherosclerosis. He says it is due to injury to artery linings resulting from blood flow disturbances. These occur at certain sites determined by the effect of the vessels on flow mechanics. It is a finding that relates to four or more other theories for the formation of atherosclerosis.

When A.H. first met Professor Rudl Altschul, with whom the effect of niacin on cholesterol was found, he spoke about this mechanical effect. Altschul's favorite hypothesis was that the inner lining, the intima, of the vessels at stressed areas did not repair itself as well. Dr. Mark D. Altschule has written that atherosclerosis occurs along the inner side of the curves in the arteries, downstream from where they divide or branch, and at points where the arteries are rigidly fixed in position by fat or by scar tissue. At these points there is a pulling or lifting effect. In response, these areas thicken, the cells change, increase, and plaque forms into a thick protuberance, which spreads in all directions along the lining of the artery. These damaged cells no longer make enough protein, creating fat instead. This is why these atherosclerotic plaques are full of cholesterol and other fats, especially the polyunsaturated fatty acids.[5,6]

Factors such as chemical poisons, viral infections, and radiation are injurious to the intima. Common poisons are carbon monoxide and cadmium from smoking, and cholesterol that has been oxidized may be especially injurious.

Mark Altschule's program for avoiding atherosclerosis is:

1. Avoid high concentrations of carbon monoxide. Smoke less and keep out of air too rich in auto exhaust.

2. Avoid obesity.
3. Avoid processed foods containing dried egg yolk or powdered milk. This we could amend by advising everyone to avoid all food artifacts—junk food.
4. Treat diabetes and high blood pressure.
5. Exercise more.

This does not mean that diet or nutrition has nothing to do with heart disease. We have no doubt that good nutrition as described in our book, *Orthomolecular Nutrition*, will decrease the incidence and prevalence of heart disease.[7]

We cannot agree with Dr. George V. Mann when he concludes that the use of nutrition to control heart disease has ended. He has, however, convincingly shown that the use of low cholesterol diets alone has not been effective. He has nothing to say about junk-free, high-fiber diets, but these have not been examined yet on as massive a scale as have been the low fat diets.[8]

Mann referred to two studies where there was no relation between diet and cholesterol blood levels, the Framingham study on 1000 subjects, and the Tecumseh study on 2000 subjects. He also referred to clinical trials where low fat diets had no effect on coronary disease but where there was an increase in cancer. Data showing an increase in consumption of polyunsaturated fats from 10.7 grams per day in 1911 to 24.2 grams per day in 1974, suggests this did not decrease coronary deaths; but at the same time, total fat intake went up from 125 grams to 158 grams.

The Carbohydrate Artifacts

Carbohydrates are primarily suppliers of energy; they are the hewers of wood and the drawers of water of the big three artifacts. In contrast to protein and fats, they are not components of body structures. Nor is much energy stored as carbohydrate. They are digested, absorbed and rapidly used for the provision of heat and energy for muscle contraction.

Carbohydrates are divided into simple and complex. Simple carbohydrates are the sugars such as glucose, fructose and galactose (monosaccharides) and sucrose, or lactose (disaccharides). All the carbohydrates are made from the simplest sugars; when digested, the carbohydrates are broken down into these sugars. They are present in small concentrations in the body. The amount in a person who has not been eating for many hours is around 80 mg of glucose per 100 ml or less than 1 percent of the blood. But this quantity is essential for life since cells depend upon glucose for life.

The body has several ways of ensuring that the amount of glucose in blood remains reasonably stable. Unfortunately, the sugar level mechanism will break down when food artifacts are consumed instead of food. Complex carbohydrates are minor components of the body. The liver and muscle tissue can store small quantities of a complex carbohydrate called *glycogen*. Complex carbohydrates are found primarily in plants. They are subdivided into those not digestible by man such as cellulose, lignin and wood, and those that are digestible such as the starches.

As with protein and fat artifacts, starch and sugar do not exist as such in nature. Foods rich in starch, such as potatoes, wheat or corn also contain all the other food constituents. In contrast, pure wheat or potato starch is a pure chemical, as are the sugars.

Carbohydrate-rich foods are safe to eat. Refined artifacts rich in carbohydrate, such as white flour, are less nutritious because so much of the other essential components has been removed. The least nutritious complex carbohydrates are the starches which are used to thicken gravies and pastries. They are, however, considerably safer than the sugars, for they are digested slowly. The released sugars are absorbed into the blood slowly so that the digestive apparatus, which must maintain steady blood glucose levels, is not swamped.

Undigestible complex carbohydrates have not been given much role in human nutrition. They were generally referred to as fiber, and most physicians either ignored them or recommended that they be avoided when they treated peptic ulcers or colitis. Low-residue diets have had a long and dishonorable history in medicine; dishonorable because lack of fiber was mainly responsible for these conditions. The low residue treatment merely made the disease worse.

The importance of fiber has been emphasized for many years by a few surgeons and physicians who were rewarded by being considered eccentrics or quacks. Recently, the work of Cleave, Campbell, and Burkitt, and a few others has brought fiber back into consideration. Dr. Burkitt, world renowned for his discovery of a type of tumor, has been indefatigable in promoting the consumption of fiber. More correctly, he has been promoting the use of foods rich in fiber content. The use of fiber alone is about as illogical as using other food artifacts alone.

Fiber serves many functions in the digestive tract. It acts as a carrier for other food components and slows down the rate of digestion. A coarse fibrous particle is degraded more slowly than a finely ground fiber free particle. As a result the products of digestion are absorbed more slowly.

Fiber acts as a carrier for many substances excreted into the gastrointestinal tract such as bile salts, heavy metals, pigments and many other substances. By binding these substances, it dilutes them and decreases their chance of harming the interior of the intestinal wall. This is how it protects against the toxic carcinogenic effect of bile salts. Fiber increases the rate at which the contents traverse the bowel. This decreases contact time between feces and intestinal wall, thus allowing less opportunity for damage to the bowel.

Fiber provides bulk. It binds several times its weight of water to form a semisolid colloid. This provides some purchase for the peristaltic waves to act upon, and increases passage rate. In the absence of fiber, feces become hard and irritating. Passage through the gut is slow and difficult, and defecation becomes painful for elderly people who suffer from constipation. Probably, laxatives are the most common over-the-counter medicine purchased by people over sixty-five. Constipation causes back pressure on the veins in the abdomen. This is the cause of varicose veins and hemorrhoids. Constant straining at stool resulting from constipation will also lead to diverticuli and diverticulosis (an inflammation of the diverticuli).

Cleave concluded that consumption of low-fiber food artifacts such as sugar, white flour and white rice leads to the Saccharine Disease. The conditions we have briefly described are merely symptoms of this Saccharine Disease. There are three main aspects of the condition:[9]

1. *A deficiency of protein that leads to peptic ulcer*—This does not mean that the daily intake of protein is too low, but means that a large intake of food artifacts is so deficient in protein that there is not enough there to bind the acid released in the stomach. If the only protein-rich meal is at dinner, while during the rest of the day, the person consumes copious quantities of coffee, soft drinks, alcohol and sugar, we have a situation where the total protein intake is adequate, but where for most of the day free acid lies in the stomach with no protein to bind it. The stomach cannot release acid, except when protein-rich foods are consumed.

2. *A surplus of rapidly digested and absorbed starchy artifacts and sugars*—This leads to obesity, diabetes, coronary disease and relative hypoglycemia. The latter condition is found in nearly every alcoholic, drug addict and obese person. It is probably present in 50 percent of our population (40 percent are obese, 5 percent are alcoholic and drug

addicts, and 3 percent are diabetic). The data which forced Cleave to the conclusion that these are symptoms of the Saccharine Disease must be read in his papers and books.

3. *A deficiency of fiber leads to constipation and its consequences such as diverticuli, ulcerative colitis and even cancer of the bowel.*

The chief villains are the sugars because they are palatable, inexpensive and ubiquitous in food artifacts. It is becoming increasingly difficult to find food (artifacts) free of sugar, and when they are found, they tend to be more expensive. Thus, the pure applesauce made by Motts and other companies is more expensive than the applesauce they make with sugar added. Also, sugar-free peanut butter costs more than ordinary peanut butter containing sugar. It is a way of selling sugar at peanut prices and an outrage.

The consumption of sucrose has remained fairly constant for the past fifty years. But the consumption of other equally toxic sugars, such as corn syrup and dextrose, has risen markedly. The total average North American sugar intake was 125.4 pounds per person in 1976. The sugar association which represents sucrose only, continues to maintain that consumption of sugar (the one it sells) has remained constant. The public doesn't realize how much hidden sugar is present in the processed food artifacts they eat. Seventy percent of all sugars consumed (88 pounds out of 125 total consumption) are obtained from processed food artifacts.

Dr. D. M. Hegsted, Professor of Nutrition, Harvard School of Public Health, at a press conference on January 14, 1977, in Washington stated,

> The diet we eat today was not planned or developed for any particular purpose. It is a happenstance related to our affluence, the productivity of our farmers and

the activities of our food industry. The risks associated with eating this diet are demonstrably large.[10]

The yearly consumption of sugars has increased enormously in the past 200 years. There has been a striking increase year by year, except for the two world wars, when the blockade decreased sugar consumption. The Germans would have been wiser not to have sunk any ships carrying sugar. Luckily, they forced the consumption of sugar to drop from about one hundred pounds to approximately sixty pounds during the first war, and caused a proportionate decrease during the second. These two periods were marked by a striking improvement in the health of the residents of Great Britain. They became healthier, both physically and mentally. This confounded the psychosomatic theorists who had confidently predicted that there would be a major increase in psychosomatic illness such as peptic ulcer and ulcerative colitis because of the stress of war.

Since the last war, the consumption of sugar has marched steadily upward. It may have peaked over the past five years and taken a downward turn now. We hope so! The officers of the companies who sell sugar-rich products have become concerned at the drop in per capita consumption of sugar, and have launched a campaign to persuade us that not only is sugar harmless, but it is positively beneficial, almost indispensable, for our health. One of their spokesmen, a well-known professor of nutrition from Harvard University, Frederick Stare, said that it would be perfectly safe for the average American to double the yearly intake of sugar—this could mean 250 pounds! The decrease in sugar intake must be credited to the increasing awareness of the public of the harmfulness of sugar. We should aim as an immediate target, a reduction to sixty pounds per person, per year, and an eventual reduction to under ten pounds.

Senator George McGovern's Select Committee on Nutrition and Human Needs, U.S. Senate, recommended that sugar consumption be reduced by 40 percent to account for 15 percent of total caloric intake. Obviously, it is impossible to reduce sugar intake too quickly, but the optimum quantity of sugar in the daily diet is zero. Every person should immediately aim for this optimum consumption, if possible. Unfortunately, just a small fraction of the public is aware of the dangers inherent in their overconsumption of sugar.

Sugar is especially harmful to the aged. Decades of sugar consumption make it almost impossible to eliminate it. It tastes good and provides a lot of calories which require little effort to consume. Often, elderly people can't chew fibrous foods and prefer soft sweet food artifacts. Sugared tea, white toast and jam are often the main meals for many of them. Whenever we see a really aged, senile person, we immediately visualize many decades of massive sugar consumption. We suggest that senility is one of the consequences of the Saccharine Disease.

Having expressed our view about the sugars, we, however, reiterate that complex polysaccharides (foods rich in starch) are nutritious, safe and important. These include whole grain cereals, vegetables and nuts. They must occupy a prominent place in our diets, unless a person is allergic to any of these foods.

We agree with the suggestions that all artifacts rich in sugars and starches be labeled with a warning that they will be harmful to your health. It should be definite and clear, and not hedged by the words "may be." Also, a new symbol for slow poison should be developed for sugar, much as the skull is used to denote more rapidly acting poisons.

References for Chapter Five

1. King, Seth S. Agriculture Department proposes new limits on "junk" food in school. *The New York Times,* July 6, 1979.

2. Consumer groups criticize "junk food" rule. *The Advocate,* July 7, 1979.

3. Shine, I. *Serendipity on St. Helena.* New York: Pergamon Press, 1970.

4. Altschul, R.; Hoffer, A.; and Stephen, J.D. Influence of nicotinic acid on serum cholesterol in man. *Archives of Biochemistry and Biophysics* 54:558 & 559, 1955.

5. Altschule, M.D. What causes your arteries to harden? *Executive Health* 10:9, 1974.

6. Altschule, M.D. Is it true what they say about cholesterol? *Executive Health* 12:11, 1976.

7. Hoffer, Abram and Walker, Morton. *Orthomolecular Nutrition,* New Canaan, Connecticut: Keats Publishing, Inc., 1978.

8. Mann, George V. Diet-heart: end of an era. *New England Journal of Medicine* 297:644-650, 1977.

9. Cleave, T.L. *The Saccharine Disease.* New Canaan, Connecticut: Keats Publishing, Inc., 1975.

10. Hegsted, D. M. *Dietary Goals for the United States.* Washington, D.C.: U.S. Government Printing Office, The Select Committee on Nutrition and Human Needs, February, 1977.

6

STRESS, OBESITY AND OTHER RISK FACTORS OF SENILITY

> *Men and women in modern society are wreaking havoc on their physical and mental health and on that of their families and friends. They seem to forget that modern life means great change, and great change is great stress, but it may be good or bad stress. . . . Some people are killed in automobile accidents or by other physical forces of destruction, but stress, though an intangible, can kill just as swiftly and surely.*
>
> —Hans Selye, Ph.D., M.D., D. Sc., "Stress: the Basis of Illness," in *Inner Balance*, 1979

A Major and Pervasive Risk Factor of Senility

AN OLD LADY is placed in a municipal nursing home by her children. An executive is named senior vice president of his company. Another loses an important sale. The mother of the bride cries during the wedding ceremony. A child packs for summer camp. A television giveaway show contestant wins a trip to Acapulco. A shopper in Chicago walks in and out of air conditioned specialty shops on Michigan Avenue during a hot summer day. A bridge toll-taker inhales the exhausts of 550 cars daily in doing his job. A motorcyclist smashes his vehicle into the rear-end of a truck and is rushed to the hospital with broken bones, a concussion and much loss of blood. A soda-fountain worker eats gobs of her ice cream concoctions continuously throughout her working hours.

What do all of these people and situations have in common? Stress. Mental, emotional, thermal, chemical or physical stress is not itself a disease or an illness. It is part of life, generated by the ever-changing life situations everyone must face. It is not necessarily bad or good. In fact, stress often is the spice of life.

Still, stress is viewed today as one of the major and pervasive problems facing the citizens of the industrialized Western countries and Japan. For too many, the stresses they live and work with result in extreme distress and the conditional precursor of many maladies such as high blood pressure, ulcers, coronary heart disease, depression, suicide, alcoholism, drug addiction, strokes, insomnia, asthma, migraine and tension headaches, kidney disease, cancer and more. It is recognized as a primary risk factor of senility and premature aging, as well.

Indeed, stress ranks among the world's worst risk factors for bringing on all kinds of health problems. People in ever-increasing numbers are affected and are being treated for a host of major and minor disabilities that appear directly related to the stress conditions under which we live. Ours is a fast-paced, success-oriented society riddled with tension, strain, anxiety, and unnatural, technological alterations in the ecology.

Industry executives and governmental bureaucrats have begun to look with alarm at the effect stress is having on corporate earnings and the national growth. Estimates by industrialists indicate that the United States alone loses more than $15 billion annually due to stress-related absenteeism, premature death, hospitalizations for disease, accidents, resignations, mental illness and low overall productivity.

What is stress? Doctors and researchers define stress as the response of the body to change—pleasant or unpleasant. If unpleasant, an individual may begin to experience physical symptoms such as pain and gastrointestinal distress or emotional symptoms such as anxiety and feelings of inadequacy or insecurity. He may become nauseous, irritable, annoyed, hesitant, pessimistic and even desperate.

In industry, one of the greatest sources of stress in any job is the threat of being fired, laid off or replaced. According to a U.S. Congressional Committee report, the 1.4 percent rise in unemployment in 1970 was associated with 1,500 suicides, 1,700 homicides, 25,000 strokes and heart and kidney deaths, 5,500 mental hospital admissions, and 800 deaths from cirrhosis of the liver, all over a five-year period.

Not all stress is job-related, of course. Often anxiety develops from a preoccupation with personal affairs: problems with a spouse or with one's children. Financial worries are a major source of stress for the elderly. These domestic difficulties can cause depression, anxiety and ultimately physical problems from psychosomatic difficulties.

In one of a series of seminars on stress and how to cope, sponsored by Riker Laboratories, Inc., F.C. Goldthorpe, M.D., Manager of Medical Education, explained that stress can be pleasant or unpleasant and changes caused by stress are not always detrimental, unless the body is unable to handle them. The key, he says, is how the body copes with stress.

Dr. Goldthorpe suggests that a person judge how well he or she is responding to stress. The body has its own alarm system which signals the body to bring the system back to normal. Without a respite from an anxiety-producing situation, the person is in danger of exhaustion and inviting serious illness—even death.

According to some researchers, personality has much to do with how well the body takes stress. People who are aggressive and striving are twice as likely to suffer coronary disease than their counterparts, who may be as competent but who lack the same obsessive drive for success.

Some new techniques evolving out of the human potential movement are being shown in workshops to help the over-achievers reduce their tendencies to self-stress. Many of the workshops are devoted to teaching these people "relaxation" exercises, some of which involve stretching out on floors and doing specific tension-relaxation exercises. Another exercise, called "instant relaxation," involves closing the eyes, taking a deep breath, holding it to the count of five and exhaling while intoning the word "relax." This exercise is designed to "neutralize," at least for the moment, the stimulus causing the stress.

Also offered in most communities are fitness programs as a means of easing tension and stress. Some programs include stress-breakers such as mountain climbing and meditation. Others consist of behavioral clinics to teach attendees how to solve personal problems, including how to cope with "midlife crisis."

Another method used to combat stress is to have individuals rate themselves on a "life change and physical ailments" scale, a list that rates by points such stressful events as the death of a spouse (100), marital separation (65), trouble with an employer (23) and so on.

The scale, it has been shown, is an early warning device for detecting oncoming illness. Nearly 90 percent of the people scoring more than 300 points during the twelve-month period that they participated in life change tests experienced a serious health problem. The following scale shown in Table I, developed by Thomas H. Holmes at the University of Washington, School of Medicine in Seattle, may predict if the amount of stress in your life will make you ill.

TABLE I

THE LIFE CHANGE SCALE

If any of these life events occurred to you in the last year, check the "Happened" column and enter its value in "Your Score" column.

Item Number	Item Value	Happened (√)	Your Score	Life Event
1	100	_____	_____	Death of your spouse
2	73	_____	_____	Divorce from your spouse
3	65	_____	_____	Separation from your spouse
4	63	_____	_____	Assigned a term in jail
5	63	_____	_____	Death of a close family member
6	53	_____	_____	Personal injury or illness (serious)
7	50	_____	_____	Embark on a new marriage
8	47	_____	_____	Fired from your steady job
9	45	_____	_____	Have a marital reconciliation
10	45	_____	_____	Enter into retirement from work
11	44	_____	_____	Change in health of a family member
12	40	_____	_____	Learn that you or your spouse is pregnant
13	39	_____	_____	Difficulties with your sexual abilities
14	39	_____	_____	Gain of a new family member
15	39	_____	_____	Have a readjustment (major) in business
16	38	_____	_____	Have a radical change in finances

17	37	_____	_____	Death of a close friend
18	36	_____	_____	Change to a different line of work
19	35	_____	_____	Alteration in number of marital arguments
20	31	_____	_____	Take on a mortgage over $10,000
21	30	_____	_____	Foreclosure of mortgage or loan
22	29	_____	_____	Responsibilities change at work
23	29	_____	_____	Son or daughter leaving home
24	29	_____	_____	Irritating trouble with in-laws
25	28	_____	_____	Recognition for outstanding achievements
26	26	_____	_____	Spouse begins to stop work
27	26	_____	_____	You begin or end schooling
28	25	_____	_____	Undergo a change in living conditions
29	24	_____	_____	You revise your personal habits
30	23	_____	_____	You experience trouble with your boss
31	20	_____	_____	Work hours or conditions are different
32	20	_____	_____	You change your residence
33	20	_____	_____	You change your school or major
34	19	_____	_____	Alterations in your recreation are marked
35	19	_____	_____	Church and club activities change
36	18	_____	_____	Social activities change exaggeratedly
37	17	_____	_____	Take out a loan or mortgage of less than $10,000
38	16	_____	_____	Your sleeping habits change
39	15	_____	_____	The number of family get-togethers change
40	15	_____	_____	Eating habits are altered
41	13	_____	_____	You go on vacation
42	12	_____	_____	The year-end Christmas holidays occur
43	11	_____	_____	You sustain a minor violation of the law

Your total score for 12 months is: _____

Stress and Malnutrition Produce Senility in Ex-POWs

We have no doubt that malnutrition alone will hasten the onset of senility or that severe unremitting stress alone will do the same, perhaps by a common mechanism. When they come together in a single elderly person, the combination is devastating to his mental and physical health. The result will surely be senility.

Severe physical and emotional stress greatly increases the loss of vitamin C and zinc, both water soluble nutrients. Most likely, there is a similar increased demand for all nutrients under stress, for stress may induce a malnutrition just as real as that which follows faulty diet. When both severe stress and malnutrition are combined, the effect is grossly magnified.

A large number of people were exposed to this combination of severe stress and malnutrition between 1935 and 1945, in Europe and the Far East. The concentration camps of Europe and the prisoner of war camps exposed millions of people to this monstrous stress from which very few have escaped. Those who survived have remained scarred physically and emotionally.

About 25 percent of the Canadian soldiers died in prison camp. In some camps housing American and English soldiers, the death rate may have been higher. When the Canadian prisoners of war (POWs) were released, the survivors were near death, having lost up to one-third of their weight. In camp, they suffered from chronic infection, from a variety of deficiency diseases of which scurvy, pellagra, and beriberi were most easily recognized, and they suffered from severe emotional and psychological shock. Many of these ex-POW's have been studied repeatedly since the end of the war. Mr. Stan Sommers has collected and published the results of these studies in the bulletin published by ex-POW's in the past two years. Physicians who were prisoners have had no difficulty recognizing the pernicious effect of incarceration, but physicians unfamiliar with the background of the ex-POW and unfamiliar with modern nutrition often fail to recognize why their patients do not get well. These doctors may fall back on the idea that their illness is psychosomatic—that they are ill because of psychological conflicts.

The delayed effects of imprisonment have been divided into two phases. The first is the stage of early after-effects from 1947 to about 1955. The second is the period of delayed after-effects. This is the phase former POWs are in now. The earlier symptoms are chronic fatigue in young adults. They find it difficult to work, but the final effects are premature aging, senility, and early death.

The cardiovascular and nervous systems were most seriously affected. Every study of the cardiovascular system shows pathology. One study of 10,000 autopsies from Dachau showed that the degree of arteriosclerosis was directly related to the duration of detention at camp. In 50 percent of all ex-POWs, half had residual psychiatric symptoms; most common were fatigue and hypersomnia.

G. W. Beebe (1975) reported in the *American Journal of Epidemiology* that ex-POWs suffered from persistent disease of the cardiovascular system, the gastrointestinal tract, the eyes; they also developed neuroses.[1] Nefsger (1970), publishing five years before in the same journal, found that ex-POWs (incarcerated by the Japanese) suffered a mortality rate 50 percent in excess of general U.S. rates for the first ten years following release. Ex-POWs (Korea) suffered a 40 percent excess rate while ex-POWs (Europe) suffered no increase except for those hospitalized for malnutrition. POWs in European camps were generally not treated as badly as those in Japanese camps. POWs (Korea) and POWs (Japan) were sicker in general; POWs (Japan) were especially marked by schizophrenia, anxiety, alcoholism and arteriosclerotic disease.[2]

These clinical investigations forced the general conclusion that these prison camps induced premature aging—the most characteristic finding. One year at war aged a soldier as much as two years of peace; one year in a camp aged a soldier the equivalent of four years at peace. A POW held by Japan for four years is at age sixty-five as old as a man of eighty-one who had never been in a prison camp. Our own estimate is one year of living in a prison camp is equal to living five years at home. Life span is decreased ten to fifteen years for war prisoners, and all POWs irrespective of country of origin suffer to the same degree. Thus, old soldiers who were held as prisoners in World War II are at high risk of turning senile.

A brief quotation from Col. E. C. Jacobs, M.D., in the *ExPOW Bulletin* for 1978, volume 35, will vividly describe the combination of malnutrition and stress:

> The Japanese army had made no preparation to feed, to transport or to house any of the Filipino-American forces. The outcome was a hundred mile "Death March" from Bataan to Camp O'Donnell at Tarlac. This forced march lasted over a period of two weeks and was made essentially without food or water, resulting in the inhumane annihilation of some 17,000 Filipino Americans and the broken bodies of all survivors. Those captives who couldn't keep up were clubbed or bayonetted in full view of the others. During the following forty months of incarceration, another 31,200 prisoners were to succumb to starvation, deficiency diseases, dysenteries, malaria and Japanese indifference and neglect. The survivors were scarred for life, and most of their lives were shortened by many years.

> A typical diet varied greatly. It was never adequate at its best being composed of a poor grade of rice and weeds. A half canteen (about 8 oz. or 160 calories) of polished rice as a thin gruel was given two or three times per day. It contained fine gravel and insects. The weeds were from water buffalo wallows. At worst, no food was given at all.

> About once a week, a water buffalo was slaughtered for 5000 to 12,000 prisoners. But after Japanese chefs removed choice cuts for themselves, each prisoner received between 4 to 16 calories of protein.[3]

The daily diet never reached 1,000 calories per day.

In our opinion, our society, even with no war conditions prevailing, affords a similar combination of stress and malnutrition to a lesser degree, and it is a major factor in hastening senility among the older population. How many senile people today had this forced upon them prematurely by the great depression of the thirties, when stress was great and many had little food to eat? We will never know unless an attempt is made to do such a retrospective study. Yet, we do know that ignorance of what is good nutrition allows near similar conditions to continue even now, not out of a lack of abundance, but from absent nutritional quality in the foods we eat.

Immunological Defenses Decrease

Aging may be due to a decrease in our immunological defenses. The immune system comprises cells which produce antibodies against foreign molecules or invaders, and the antibodies inactivate the invading cells. With age, fewer antibodies are produced, making us more vulnerable to infections and cancer. It is also believed that our cells can misrecognize our own cells as foreign and attack them with antibodies. Auto-immune diseases are degenerative diseases associated with aging.

Slow acting viruses may be present which require decades for their destructive effect to occur. The virus may so alter body cells that they seem foreign and are attacked by antibodies, thus hastening aging.

The brain itself may control aging by its regulation of hormones. Over the past two decades, it has become clear that the pituitary and hypothalamic hormones are involved in brain activity and have an effect upon behavior. The behavior of rats becomes abnormal when their pituitary gland is removed. It is also abnormal in rats who have hereditary diabetes insipidus where vasopressin is not available. Giving them ACTH or vasopressin restores normal behavior.

In hypophysectomized rats, behavior becomes normal when they are given fragments of ACTH, lipotropin and vasopressin which have no hormone properties. Neuroleptics related to ACTH have a short term effect on behavior. Those related to vasopressin have a long term effect.

Vasopressin is involved in memory, and, of course, failing memory is a main characteristic of senility. Rats with a genetic defect in the synthesis of vasopressin are inferior in retaining active and passive avoidance behavior. They do not remember as well. Vasopressin appears to promote memory consolidation or retrieval.

De Wied and his colleagues have reviewed the evidence that vasopressin is involved in memory. A single injection of arginine-8-vasopressin increased resistance to extinction of a pole-jumping avoidance response in rats. Smaller amounts placed in the ventricles of the brain were as effective. Vasopressin, the antidiuretic hormone, is a peptide bound to a protein, neurohypophysen II, which is stored in granules.[4,5]

De Wied concluded "Findings so far indicate the existence of neuropeptides which affect learning, memory and motivation," other neuropeptides have opiate-like activity and affect sleep, thirst, aggression, and the development of tolerance and physical dependence.[6]

Legros and colleagues found that neurophysen blood levels decreased in people after age fifty. This is an index of a decrease in the activity of the neurohypophysis. They tested the effect of inhaling vasopressin on memory. Twelve subjects were given 16 IU of vasopressin daily, one puff to each nostril three times per day. Eleven were given placebo. Those on vasopressin did better on attention, concentration, motor rapidity and memory tests.[7]

Oliveros reported four patients with amnesia responded to vasopressin. The one alcoholic responded least well.

The remaining three suffering from post traumatic retrograde and antero grade amnesia responded better.[8]

Obesity and Hypoglycemia

We have stated that average Americans and Canadians consume over 125 pounds of simple sugars per year, and their intake of sucrose—table sugar—has remained constant for the past fifty years. The commercial sugar association makes much of this leveling off in its papers and press releases. What they ignore is that other sugars such as corn syrup and dextrose have been consumed at an ever increasing rate. The latter are usually hidden in various foods where they are least expected such as mayonnaise, soups, crackers and so on. Most of the patients placed on a sugar-free diet are astonished when they monitor their sugar intake by what they read on the labels of boxes and cans they buy. There is an undeniable relationship between the consumption year by year of these toxic levels of the sugars and the Saccharine Disease. We have already described the manifestations of the Saccharine Disease, but we have neglected to comment on the combined effect of sugar and salt in our diet.

Dr. D.J.R. Rowe (*Canadian Medical Association Journal*, October 1978) is concerned about the additive effect of salt and sugar. Canadians and Americans eat an average of 10 grams of salt (⅓ of an ounce) per day, while only about 0.5 grams is required. More than 2 grams per day is dangerous for hypertensives. It is generally accepted that high blood pressure results from a disturbance of the equilibrium between noradrenalin and the sympathetic nervous system. Also recognized is the increased sensitivity and responsiveness to angiotensin II and noradrenaline of the vascular smooth muscle. The latter feature is associated with a disturbance in arterial cation content or ratios secondary to an excessive *sodium* intake in predisposed persons or to a mild increase in mineral corticoid activity.

Hypertension and obesity are related as they are to pathological changes in the brain leading to senility. A number of societies have normal blood pressure, which does not increase with age, including the Caracas Indians, Thais, Ethiopians, African bushmen and Uganda nomads. They consume one-tenth of the salt of average Americans.[9]

A recent study showed that in monkeys, either sugar or salt increased blood pressure, but when both were given together, the effect was much greater. Since high blood pressure is an important risk factor for cerebrovascular disease, it must also be a high risk factor for senility.

Excessive sugar consumption is associated with obesity. Obesity can usually be directly related to the sugar tolerance where it causes reactive hypoglycemia (relative hypoglycemia). For this reason, biochemical changes related to obesity may not be unique to the obese condition, but to the high intake of sugars. In our opinion, excessive intake of sugars, obesity and hypoglycemia are risk factors for senility, even when blood pressure is not elevated.

In a recent review, Dr. A. Angel (*Canadian Medical Association Journal,* December 1978) summarized the changes found in the obese. As a result of overeating, adipose mass made up of large round fat-containing cells supported by collagen and fed by many capillaries and sympathetic nerves increases markedly. These cells are more active in fat metabolism in the obese. Plasma fat concentrations are elevated with the most common abnormality being an increase in triglycerides. Sugar and alcohol excess drives the liver to make large amounts of fatty acids which leads to increased triglyceride levels. Low density lipoproteins (LDL) are the main cholesterol transport particles in plasma, and they increase in obesity. High density lipoproteins (HDL) are made by the liver. They have antiarteriosclerotic properties. Several studies have shown an inverse relationship between plasma HDL and coronary artery disease. Human adipose cells degrade HDL in significant amounts.[10]

Obese people have more cholesterol, most of it stored in

the fat cells. Daily cholesterol production is increased in proportion to the degree of obesity.

Medical complications of obesity include cardiovascular disease arising from high blood pressure, diabetes, reduced plasma HDL and hypercholesterolemia. Cerebrovascular disease and stroke occur more often in the obese.

Many elderly people enjoy an alcoholic drink, often with a sugar-containing mix. It relaxes them in the evening and later they use it to induce sleep, but this is a potent mixture for causing hypoglycemia, a main risk factor for senility.

Dr. S.J.D. O'Keefe and Dr. V. Marks (*The Lancet,* June, 1977) measured the effect of alcohol mixed with tonic in ten young subjects on blood sugar levels. Each one drank gin and tonic containing over 1½ ounces of alcohol (50 grams) and 60 grams of sucrose. This caused more profound hypoglycemia than alcohol alone. Mood changes correlated with blood alcohol and sugar levels: One hour after drinking, the subjects felt pleasantly inebriated when blood sugar was at its peak: in a few cases, when alcohol peak occurred after blood glucose began to fall, subjects became depressed.[11]

Nutrient Deficiency and Dependency

Soon after the vitamin concept was established early in the twentieth century, nutritionists began to describe deficiency diseases. If the diet lacked thiamine, the deficiency disease, beriberi arose; deficiency of niacin caused pellagra; deficiency of ascorbic acid brought on scurvy; and lack of vitamin D created the condition of rickets. Much later, it was recognized that some individuals suffer from the same problems because their requirement for the vitamin is so very much greater—even a diet adequate for most is inadequate for them. This could have been called a "relative dependency" since the problem is mainly in the increased requirement for the nutrient and not in the food supply.

Of course, there is no sharp demarcation and all individuals must be somewhere on a continuum ranging from those who remain well on quantities which would be inadequate for the majority, to those whose needs may be one hundred to one thousand times as great.

A large number of reactions crop up between the time the nutrient is ingested and its final interaction in the cell. The reason for dependency may reside in any one or more of these reactions, including:

1. Destruction or binding of the vitamin in the intestinal tract by certain foods, bacteria or parasites, and
2. A defect in the absorptive capacity of the intestine due to chronic use of laxatives, chronic disease, following surgical removal of portions or genetic or acquired defect in those areas which have a specific absorptive capacity such as for vitamin B-12. Malnutrition may reduce absorption and inadequate fat intake will decrease absorption of fat soluble vitamins for example.
3. Before the B vitamins, thiamine, riboflavin, niacin, pyridoxine, and vitamin B-12 become functional, they must be incorporated into larger molecules called coenzymes. There could be a block or defect in the coenzyme formation reactions. Increasing the amount of vitamin in solution would drive the formation reaction toward synthesis of more coenzyme.
4. Vitamins may not be conserved as well or may be destroyed too quickly.
5. There may be an increased destruction due to stress. Thus during any physical or mental stress, there is a marked increase in destruction of vitamin C.

Vitamin dependency may be genetic (inherited) or acquired. The permanent ill health of the ex-POWs previously discussed is an example of a vitamin B-3 dependency acquired by severe stress and malnutrition. Perhaps they were also made dependent on other vitamins.

Pellagrologists were physicians who specialized in pellagra. Once it was shown pellagra was cured by vitamin B-3, the need for pellagrologists vanished. There are none around today in North America, although there are still a few in India researching this disease. Early pellagrologists were surprised that chronic pellagrins required up to 600 mg. of vitamin B-3 per day, while pellagrins who had been ill for short periods of time only required doses under 50 mg. This huge requirement (for that era) violated the definition of a vitamin as something required in minute quantities. They made no attempt to explain this.

Trace elements are also required in different quantities. There is no scientific reason why there should not be dependencies on zinc or other water soluble minerals; this would be less probable for toxic metals. Since all nutrients are required, one nutrient cannot be more important than another. For any individual, however, the one or more nutrients that he is dependent on will be relatively more important. The rest may be easily available from food, but those on which he is dependent will be required as extra food supplements.

We strongly believe that nutrient deficiencies and dependencies play a major role in the development of senility. This means there are as many types of senility as there are dependencies or deficiencies. Grey hair is one of the manifestations of aging. For some people, taking large doses of vitamin E restores their original hair color. One of us (AH) began to grey over ten years ago, but to his surprise, 800 IU of vitamin E restored his hair color. For other individuals, other nutrients will do the same, because there is no general relationship of one vitamin to hair color or to senility.

In our experience, some of the vitamins play a more important role than others when taken in orthomolecular doses, but all must be provided in optimal doses. In the next chapter, we will describe in detail the various vitamins necessary as an antisenility nutrient formula. You can take nutrients to age without senility.

References for Chapter Six

1. Beebe, G. W. Follow-up studies of World War II and Korean War prisoners, II, morbidity, disability, and maladjustments. *American Journal of Epidemiology* 101:400-422, 1975.

2. Negsfer, M. D. Follow-up studies of World War II and Korean prisoners, I, study plan and mortality findings. *American Journal of Epidemiology* 91:123-138, 1970.

3. Jacobs, E. C. Residuals of Japanese prisoner-of-war thirty years later. *Ex POW Bulletin* 35:15-18, 1978.

4. De Wied, D. Behavioral effects of intraventricularly administered vasopressive and vasopresser fragments. *Life Sciences* 19:685-690, 1976.

5. De Wied, D.; Van Wimers, M. A.; Greidanus, T. B.; Bohus, B.; Urban, I; and Gispen, W. H. Vasopressers and memory consolidations, perspectives in brain research. *Progress in Brain Research.* Ed. Corner, M. A. and Swaab, D. F. Vol 45. Elsevier, Holland: North Holland Biomedical Press, 1976.

6. De Wied, D. Peptides and behavior. *Life Sciences* 20:195-204, 1977.

7. Legros, J. J.: Gilot, P.; Seron, X.; Claessens, J.; Adam, A.; Moeglèn, J. M.; Audibert, A.; and Bercher, D. Influence of vasopressers on learning and memory. *The Lancet* 1:41-42, 1978.

8. Oliveros, J. C.; Jandali, M.K.: Timsit-Bethier, M.; Remy, R.; Benghezal, A.; Audibert, A.; and Moeglen, J. M. Vasopressers in amnesia. *The Lancet* 1:42, 1978.

9. Rowe, D.J.R. Salt and sugar in the diet. *Canadian Medical Association Journal* 119:786-790, 1978.

10. Angel, A. Pathophysiologic changes in obesity. *Canadian Medical Association Journal* 119:1401-1406, 1978.

11. O'Keefe, S.J.D. and Marks, V. Lunchtime gin and tonic, a cause of reactive hypoglycemia. *The Lancet* 1:1286·1288, 1977.

7

THE ANTISENILITY VITAMINS

If you had three wishes, what would they be?

1. Not to survive my intelligence; in other words, to be able to write effectively and thoughtfully for as long as I live—however long that may be.

2. To cause no sorrow when I leave this life; in other words, to have all those who both love me and survive me to be so glad I have lived effectively and happily that they will feel no need to mourn.

3. And most of all—to live long enough to see humanity make the crucial decisions for survival; in other words, to die knowing that civilization will survive after all into the 21st century, and for as long thereafter as is possible.

—Isaac Asimov, *The New York Times*, May 15, 1977

The Woman Who Outlived Her Intelligence

MARTHA BLOOM, the mother of my wife, Joan Walker, was a woman to whom everyone who knew her and some who only knew of her came for advice. She had a wisdom to share, strength to support, and serenity to calm the most anxious friend, neighbor, or family member. People flocked to the apartment in Jamaica, Queens, New York where Martha Bloom lived to find answers to their questions or assistance with their burdens. She offered love and caring, and they came to her for knowledge on the fulfillment of their personal needs.

She was a stable force in the lives of seventeen brothers and sisters belonging to her husband Julius and herself. They all sought the wise counsel that came from her alert mind. Self-educated, but dispensing a home-spun philosophy brought from eastern Europe when she was a very young woman, Mrs. Bloom increased her knowledge with much reading of the classics and nonfiction books.

She owned a mental storehouse of medical information and used to live in the most natural way possible in an urban environment. She fed her immediate family fresh foods, rarely used canned goods, and cooked delicious meals with food aplenty for anyone who might drop in. I remember how Mom Bloom enjoyed watching me shovel in the victuals at her table. She also was an exponent of exercise. The result was an abundant health for those who followed her example.

The world caved in for Martha Bloom, however, when Julius, in his seventy-second year, was struck by cancer and had a lung removed. For more than a year, she nursed him while he underwent chemotherapy and radiation therapy, but the unrelenting cancer metastasized. Laboring under severe stress, she did everything possible to make her husband well—all to no avail. He died and left Martha at age sixty-seven to live alone. This stressful event was almost unendurable, and she became ill herself.

Her hair turned white in that unbearable year, and she tried to find comfort in her four children, their children and the coming of great-grandchildren. But over time, stress piled upon stress—in the form of financial worries, fear for her own safety in a city that is an asphalt jungle, the deaths of sisters and brothers one by one, and a lingering, brooding sense of loss that never left her. "I want to be with Julius," she said, and meant it.

Worst of all was an attack of hiatus hernia that forced her to adopt an unnatural eating program of soft processed foods she wasn't use to. *Hiatus hernia* is the rupture or protrusion of part of the stomach through the esophageal opening of the diaphragm. Mrs. Bloom, following her physician's prescription, had to give up the fresh fruits and fresh vegetables she was accustomed to eating. The dead foods—white bread, white rice, softened crackers, gruel and other mushy substances, and antiacid medicines —deadened the symptoms and deadened the brain. The soft diet was another form of stress.

My mother-in-law lost weight, found less energy, stopped her regular exercise program of long walks, and began looking to a plethora of doctors for help. Each one gave her a different drug prescription to relieve her various symptoms, treating what they called "old age." Nothing seemed to help, however, and at seventy-five, this formerly active and healthy woman regressed rapidly into the familiar signs of senescence.

At first, senility manifested itself with her inability to put words together during conversations; she forgot the names of her grandchildren; lost the trend of ideas; couldn't read words on a page because of rapidly diminishing vision. Even television, which Mrs. Bloom once held in disdain, flashed before her as darkened images that slowly became mere shadows. She slept a great deal and withdrew into herself more and more. She remembered happenings in the distant past but not what she ate for breakfast that same morning—or if she had eaten breakfast at all. Often she actually forgot to eat and began to show the effects of neglect.

Her children realized that although it would be a blow to her pride, she could not live alone any longer. Mom Bloom preferred not to give up her home and move in with one of her children, so they hired a nurse to move in with her instead.

Also, two daughters took her to visit Francis Ferrer, M.D., of New York City. In response to new journalistic information just filtering in to me relating to orthomolecular nutrition (before I met Dr. Hoffer and the Academy of Orthomolecular Psychiatry), my wife and one of her sisters,

Adele Weitzberg, sought and found an orthomolecular nutritionist. Dr. Ferrer prescribed a wide assortment of nutritional supplements and assured us that taking them routinely would help Mom Bloom keep her thoughts together.

The nutrients did seem to accomplish their purpose when the daughters managed to get their mother to swallow the capsules and tablets on a regular basis. But she considered any kind of pills like the "medicine" she had been against taking her whole life. She fought every swallow. She flushed the supplements down the toilet when her nurse wasn't watchful. It was this cantankerousness and the vituperative arguments connected with it that finally forced her companion to quit.

Mom Bloom's son and three daughters were frantic to find another person to stay with the senile eighty-year-old lady, but there was no one to be found. They took turns living in their mother's apartment. Joan's weekly roundtrip visits from our Connecticut home to Jamaica, New York stretched into overnight stays. The four children had to find a permanent arrangement and while they searched for it, they renewed giving her antisenility nutrients although by now her senile syndrome was very well established.

Indeed, Mom Bloom's mind was hardly functioning at all. She couldn't hold any thought or put a few words together in a full sentence. She couldn't walk alone; fell frequently; was unable to dress herself; could not feed herself; and made no expression of wants or needs. Very rarely did she comprehend what was said to her. She mumbled in Yiddish, a reversion to her original language, spoken in Russia almost three quarters of a century before. Lingering in some other time and place, she seemed even beyond recent past experiences. She gave no responses to any direct approach about some family occurrence that should have been meaningful.

The children found a place for Mom Bloom in an

excellent convalescent hospital that catered to her kind of senescence. She received the best nursing and medical care that orthodox medicine had available. But the hospital administration was so traditional in its methods that orthomolecular nutrition using dietary supplementation with vitamins and minerals was turned down as bordering on "quackery." Although Joan and Adele were persistent and tried to persuade the authorities to give the nutrients a chance, no one in the hospital would take it on themselves to give my mother-in-law vitamins and minerals on a regular basis. Kind attendants who might have indulged the daughters were too frightened of placing their jobs in jeopardy.

The dietary supplements were abandoned although Adele and Joan believe they would have saved their mother had she been given them consistently. The nutrients never had an opportunity to work. At home, the patient in her mental illness considered those pills poison and refused to swallow them. In the hospital, the authorities regarded nutrients against senility as some kind of black magic. They laughed at nutritional therapy and declared Martha Bloom's senility irreversible. No provision could be made at the nursing home by her daughters to continue the patient on dietary supplementation.

At eighty-three Mom Bloom finally died under the observing eyes of the gentle nurses and the astute physicians. I can only wonder why, with all the kind, considerate, and wonderful acts they performed for her in keeping her clean, dressing her, spoon-feeding her, trying to get her to respond to some outside stimulus, they absolutely refused to put a few vitamin pills in her mouth and help her swallow them with a little water? What would have been so wrong in that?

I believe that ten or fifteen years ago if any of her children or their mates had understood the science of orthomolecular nutrition, we might have saved my mother-in-law from the living death of senility. She would not have outlived her intelligence. But the family did not know. I did not know then. Mom Bloom is now gone for two years, and I love the memory of what she had been.

Orthomolecular Nutrition for Senility

The nursing hospital in which Martha Bloom died violated the first rule of Claude Bernard, the great 19th century French physiologist, whose researches were concerned with the pancreas, the glycogenic function of the liver, and the discovery of the vasomotor system. Dr. Bernard said that any treatment program which may be of benefit to the patient, and which is not harmful, is obligatory to be used.

Furthermore, in a paraphrase of Claude Bernard's rule, we have concluded with regard to the specific treatment of senility that any procedure therapeutic for it should be even more effective in its prevention. The treatment of presenility or premature aging is already a preventive program since it avoids or slows down any further deterioration of the mind.

The program of nutrition against senility which follows in this and other chapters is derived from our experience with presenile and senile patients, interviews with orthomolecular physicians, and a search of the scientific literature. Because individuals are so variable, we will lay down general rules and descriptions of the various nutrients and merely suggest the desirable dosages. Realize that nutrition is the most important aspect of treatment for the senile, and there is no good substitute for nutritious food. As we pointed out in Chapter Six, unfortunately the nutrition in food is largely lost by processing. Consequently, we must suggest supplements in the form of vitamin and mineral tablets, capsules, and powders.

Senility is a disease, not a way of life and not inevitable. In most cases, it is due to chronic malnutrition, for which society, the food processors, and the consumer share the blame. However, orthomolecular nutrition is the correction, and orthomolecular nutrition is enhanced with the use of food supplements, beginning with the various vitamins which we shall discuss one by one but not necessarily in the order of their importance.

Thiamine (Vitamin B-1)

The classical thiamine deficiency state, beriberi, causes psychiatric and neurologic symptoms which, if they occurred in an older person, could easily be diagnosed as senile changes. Thiamine is essential for the metabolism of sugar. When large quantities of sugar are consumed, the body's metabolism tends to increase its own demand for the vitamin in the same way alcohol increases the demand for it. Alcohol and sugar are closely related in their causal response from the body.

In contrast to carbohydrate-rich foods which carry enough thiamine as a component to metabolize the sugar in the whole food, sugar-rich artifacts carry none or too little thiamine. The consumption of sugar artifacts creates a net deficit in the vitamin economy of the body. It is a condition similar to *Wernicke-Korsakoff syndrome,* the partial destruction of the brain resulting from a lack of thiamine in chronic alcoholics.

The Wernicke-Korsakoff syndrome was first described by Korsakoff as being present in people with a long history of alcoholism.

It is also present in people who have not been alcoholic, but there is an unfortunate tendency to consider only alcoholism as a cause. Since early Korsakoff's syndrome is treated with large doses of thiamine, those cases who are not recognized because they are not alcoholics will not be treated adequately. Bowerman (1978) recently reviewed Korsakoff's three pages containing the disease's original clinical description. He was particularly struck by the association of mental and neurological symptoms.[1] Researchers have concluded that what was considered two syndromes, Korsakoffs and Wernicke, were in fact one, Wernicke-Korsakoff syndrome. Korsakoff's syndrome emphasized the mental symptoms and Wernicke's, the neurological symptoms.

The mental symptoms include anxiety and depression, obsessive thinking, confusion, defective memory, especially for recent events, time distortion, emotional liability, irritability, agitation and sometimes confabulation. This certainly is not unlike the mental changes of the senile person. Wernicke-Korsakoff can be caused by infection, cerebral hemorrhage and post surgical complications usually within twenty-four hours.

The symptoms wax and wane and the patient may cover them up successfully for a long time, but symptoms reappear when slight or severe stress is placed upon the person. These include surgery, accidents, injuries, an extra job, unusual work and other stressors. Memory problems are the first to appear. In some, symptoms have been present many years as a form of minimal brain dysfunction. At times, these patients have had periods of hyperactivity and drive which they found advantageous. Bowerman concludes,

> Not only has alcohol become an artifact because of the prominence of the findings in the alcoholics, but also perhaps because the alcoholic has a pronounced mental and physical response to life's stresses for which he uses alcohol as self-medication. Thus what was thought to be an etiology is rather self-medication for the condition.

It is possible that many senile people are simply examples of Wernicke-Korsakoff disease where the additional stresses of age have precipitated another outburst of symptoms. Many seniles do have to a milder degree the same symptoms found in alcoholic Wernicke-Korsakoff syndrome (W-K syndrome).

Thiamine deficiency and/or perhaps thiamine dependency is the main cause of this condition. Alcoholics consume large quantities of alcoholic beverages, and thiamine is essential for the metabolism of alcohol as it is for sugar and carbohydrate in general. Since many alcoholics cannot afford to eat and also maintain their alcoholic intake, and since alcohol provides calories, there is a decrease in the consumption of food containing vitamins and minerals. Unless the alcoholic makes a special effort to eat very nutritious food (and few do), there inevitably must be a deficiency of all vitamins and minerals.

An editorial in *The New York Times* written by Brandon Centerwall, a medical student at the University of California, San Diego, makes an excellent recommendation to which we adhere. Why not put thiamine in beer, wine, whiskey and other alcoholic beverages? Wernicke-Korsakoff syndrome can be prevented—simply add the vitamin to all liquor. It is stable, does not change a drink's flavor, and is known to be safe. It seems a logical additive in all liquor, wine and beer to reverse the symptoms of the syndrome.[2]

The W-K syndrome may appear in those who are thiamine dependent. Men and women who consume large quantities of refined sugars may be just as vulnerable. If this is an important factor, we can expect to see a significant increase in W-K syndrome among the younger generation when they reach their sixties and seventies. The massive consumption of food artifact has occurred in the past two decades. We are just beginning to see the children of the first generation of heavy junk consumers. This generation may well provide the first surge in the incidence of senility in about forty to fifty years. If you want to protect yourself against this senile occurrence, the correct thiamine intake is 250 mg a day in divided doses.

Niacin-Nicotinic Acid (Vitamin B-3)

Nicotinic acid (known medically as niacin) and nicotinamide (niacinamide) are antipellagra vitamins incorporated into the coenzyme nicotinamide-adenine dinucleotide

(NAD). A derivative of vitamin B-3 in nature exists in this coenzyme form or is bound to the tissues as nucleotides. Sometimes it is so firmly bound, the vitamin can't be released in the body. This is the situation with corn and accounts for one of the reasons corn diets frequently are predisposed to pellagra.

It is likely that the deficiency of any essential nutrient, if continued for a long time, will hasten the onset of senility, but a reduced intake of niacin especially illustrates the truth of this statement. Its deficiency seems most responsible for a rapid development of the senile syndrome.

NAD participates in a large number of reactions requiring transport of electrons or oxidation reduction reactions. This is such an important enzyme that the body has developed several methods for ensuring that it is retained. NAD is made from vitamin B-3, originating from the amino acid L-tryptophan and is also made from the vitamin present in food. Finally when the pyridine molecule is recycled in the body, NAD is split into nicotinamide, some of which is converted into nicotinic acid, and pyridine is incorporated into NAD. This is called the *pyridine nucleotide cycle*.

When there is too little vitamin B-3 in the food, the deficiency disease pellagra develops. Pellagra is a chronic deteriorating illness which invariably leads to death unless the vitamin B-3 is replaced. The early stages of pellagra produce depression, anxiety, and fatigue.

For a while, pellagrologists debated whether to include early pellagra among the neuroses. It certainly produces a characteristic neurotic reaction, and later it produces a psychotic reaction—usually a schizophrenic syndrome. If the disease progresses, the clinical syndrome becomes an organic psychosis which, like all organic psychoses, resembles the senile psychoses.

Pellagra, the preterminal disease, is seldom found in our society. The fortification of flour with nicotinamide provides most people with just enough vitamin to protect them against this. Or does it? The definition of pellagra depends so heavily on a deficiency of vitamin B-3 in our diet, that if a similar disease occurred in the presence of normal amounts of vitamin B-3, no nutritionist or physician would call it pellagra. Furthermore, most physicians and nutritionists have accepted the assumption that our diet is so good that even the idea of any substantial proportion of our population suffering from a deficiency is unthinkable.

A proportion of any population requires much more vitamin than the majority of people—to the degree that even a diet completely healthy for most would be inadequate in this factor for some. These people are said to have a vitamin dependency, which we have already mentioned. But to clarify again: *having a vitamin dependency means that for this person there is a relative deficiency of this vitamin.* It does not differ in any way from the deficiency disease pellagra—the pellagra caused by a dependency may differ from the deficiency pellagra since the dependent person will be more chronic and will have other metabolic processes of which the vitamin B-3 dependency is the result.

I first realized in 1953 that nicotinic acid could help patients with organic brain damage of a milder sort as takes place in senility. Humphry Osmond and I had already started our experiments using large doses of nicotinic acid for treating schizophrenia. I was familiar with its use and its relative safety. One day I flew to a small town in Saskatchewan to spend a day examining patients referred to the public health center by local physicians. One of my patients was a middle-aged woman who had completed a series of electroconvulsive therapy (ECT) one month before. She was referred again because her memory was so awful she could not function.

There is no doubt that post ECT amnesia is a measure of some cerebral pathology. Forunately, it is transient and very rarely leaves a permanent memory defect except that the memory of events occurring during the ECT may not return.

In 1953, there was no treatment for post ECT amnesia, but I started the woman on nicotinic acid, 3 grams per day without any conviction it would help, although I was certain it would do no harm. One month later, when I saw her again, she was normal. She and her husband reported that one week after starting the niacin treatment, her memory cleared. Since then, for 22 years, I have observed on several hundred patients given ECT that there is much less residual memory defect when they take nicotinic acid concurrently and after the series of ECT. In most cases, the nicotinic acid can be discontinued unless there are other reasons why it should be used. The memory defect will not come back.

Double blind experiments are not required to show the antisenility effect of nicotinic acid. The original idea for using the type of experiment called "double blind" arose as a way of dealing with diseases which vary exceedingly such as the common cold or some forms of arthritis. When diseases come and go, one can always say that what appears to be a therapeutic response may simply be a natural recovery. Senility has a generally progressive downhill course, and no one has reported spontaneous recoveries from it. When a few patients do recover with any treatment, one must accept that the treatment is effective until further experiments prove the results were spurious. From our own experience alone, we are convinced that nicotinic acid is very effective if it is started before the senility is too well established. We will therefore not discuss this any further but will present a number of explanations which account for the vitamin's antisenility property.

Niacin Lowers Blood Fats, Cholesterol and Triglycerides

For most people, at least 3 grams of niacin must be used before there is any significant effect in lowering blood fats.

Sometimes as much as 6 grams is required. The slow release preparations are more effective. In a few experiments, we found that 0.5 grams of slow release (SR) niacin was more effective than 6 grams for the same person. Niacinamide has no effect. The reason for this difference is still unknown.

Niacin was one of four compounds studied in the $40 million Coronary Drug Project which involved 55 research clinics and 8,341 patients, all of whom had recovered from a heart attack. Two of the compounds, estrogen and dextro-thyroxine, were discontinued before the study was completed because of a slight increase in mortality. The remaining two, niacin and clofibrate, were continued until termination in 1975. The use of clofibrate for treating coronary disease was not supported by the results. About niacin, the investigators concluded, "It may be slightly beneficial in protecting persons to some degree against recurrent nonfatal myocardial infarctions."

Long before this coronary drug study began, Prof. E. Boyle had placed about 160 similar patients on niacin and followed them carefully for over ten years, giving each one individual attention. An equivalent group not given niacin, a control group, if one were run, would have lost sixty patients in that time by death. Only six died. Boyle concluded niacin had reduced the mortality by about 90 percent. He was one of the consultants to the massive niacin study.

Boyle pointed out in a private discussion with us that in the double blind coronary study, the individual attention to each patient on niacin was not given. A large number of physicians were involved who had no particular experience or interest in it. In addition, when patients complained of side effects, the medication was discontinued. However, the total number of patients who had started on niacin were used in the final calculations, even though they may have been on it for only a portion of the total study. Recently a re-evaluation of some of the published data showed that the original reporters had neglected certain other data which showed niacin to have a more positive effect than is suggested by the conclusion quoted above.

Finally, since Atromid has come off so badly in the recent English study, there is only one substance left which can reliably lower fats in the blood. (There are of course other ways of lowering fat levels using dietary methods.) Niacin is the only safe hypolipidemic substance and will be useful in treating those with an inherited tendency for high blood cholesterol levels. These people often suffer heart attacks between the ages of thirty and fifty.

Prof. R. Altschul in his book reviewed the evidence that niacin taken over a period of several years could reverse some of the arteriosclerotic pathology in blood vessels.

Recent studies suggest niacin may be valuable in treating recent heart attacks. Fatty acids can interfere with the ability of the heart to use glucose. They may disturb heart rhythm leading to abnormal, potentially fatal, arrhythmia. A heart attack is accompanied by an increase in free fatty acids in the blood. Apparently any serious stress can do the same. The fatty acids are mobilized from fat depots by the secretion of adrenalin. Niacin prevents the release of the fatty acids while it does not interfere with the release of adrenalin. It stabilizes the fatty acids in the cells which store the fat. In one study on ten normal subjects, niacin stopped the interference of fatty acids in heart muscle metabolism. In another study, a niacin analogue which also lowered free fatty acids in blood, a similar beneficial effect was observed during heart attacks. Men given this substance within five hours of the onset of a heart attack had fewer serious heart arrhythmias.

Antisludging Effect

Sludging is the term applied to red blood cells which do not float freely in blood but which adhere to each other, as we described previously. Capillaries are so small that the red cells pass through in single file. When two or more red blood cells adhere or stick to each other, they cannot traverse the capillaries. These capillaries therefore carry plasma only, with no red blood cells. The tissues fed by these capillaries suffer from anoxia. If many cells are sludged, large areas of tissues are deprived of oxygen.

Anoxic areas are probably more susceptible to tissue death, to small hemorrhages or small infarcts. Preventing sludging will therefore prevent or reverse senile changes caused by sludging.

Nicotinic acid apparently acts by increasing the electronegative charge on each cell. Cells are better able to repel each other.

Whether it acts this way or not, there is little doubt that the vitamin has antisludging properties. We have seen many patients whose faces appeared pallid and sickly, who complained of chronic fatigue, memory failure, depression, and anxiety. These are the patients most apt to suffer from sludging. After a few months on nicotinic acid therapy, their skin becomes clear, healthy, and of a normal color. At the same time, their fatigue and other symptoms are diminished or gone entirely.

Restoration of Coenzyme One (NAD)

With a deficiency of the NAD enzyme, most reactions would be diminished, since the brain must have a steady flow of energy. Megadoses of nicotinic acid probably restore coenzyme function.

The Niacin Effect on Peripheral Vascular Disease

Two serious peripheral vascular diseases, chilblains and Raynaud's disease, respond to adequate amounts of niacin. Chilblains is a painful reddening of fingers, toes or ears following exposure to cold. Raynaud's disease consists of intermittent attacks of blanching or blueness of the fingers, often with pain, caused by cold or emotional distress. We have seen the beneficial effect of niacin on Raynaud's disease and now consider this an indication for using niacin.

Tetranicotinoylfructose is split in the gut, slowly releasing niacin. In this reaction, it resembles linodil, inositol hexaniocotinate. Studies with the tetra derivative showed that it increased blood flow in the extremities. In a joint Australian-Scottish study, it was concluded that vitamin B-3 should be valuable for treating conditions such as Raynaud's disease and chilblains.

Arthritis

William Kaufman, M.D., of Stratford, Connecticut, began to use vitamin B-3 in gram doses for treating arthritis and found it very effective for most cases. Using a precise method for measuring joint mobility, he developed an index with 100 as the maximum or normal score. Severely arthritic patients had scores below 50. When treated, the scores all increased. For older people, it increased 12 points within two months. For some, it increased 31 points. Before becoming aware of Kaufman's prior discovery, one of us (AH) had made the same clinical observation in 1954. Since then, most orthomolecular physicians have observed the same antiarthritic beneficial effect. The two books written by Kaufman are available from him directly at 395 A. Ottawa Lane, Stratford, CT 06497.

Niflumic acid, a derivative of niacin, was found to be as effective as endomethacin, one of the widely used drugs for rheumatoid arthritis. A larger study in Norway showed it was effective and well tolerated over a long period. At the University of Lund, Sweden, it was found to be as effective in osteoarthritis as endomethacin.

Some of the common symptoms in ex-POWs are arthritic limitation of movement, with pain. These symptoms respond particularly quickly to vitamin B-3. The antiarthritic properties of vitamin B-3 certainly place it among the valuable antisenile compounds as well when given in the appropriate dosage.

The Antisenility Dosage of Vitamin B-3

The earlier a person starts on vitamin supplementation with nicotinic acid or nicotinamide, the less dosage is required. We would recommend the following doses for people who do not feel that whole foods alone provide adequate nutrition. The closer you are to the age of senility, even if not senile, the more you should be taking preventive measures.

Age 20–29	100 mg niacin after each meal
30–39	300 mg niacin after each meal
40–49	500 mg niacin after each meal
50 and over	1000 mg niacin after each meal

You can start with a low dose and gradually work up or begin with the full dose, but beware of an initial flush. If the flush is too irritating, you should start a low dosage and work up to the larger one slowly over a few weeks. A person needing the higher dosage generally will have the fewest side effects when he begins to use the vitamin.

Nicotinamide (niacinamide) may work just as well if it is started many years before the possible onset of senility. But the closer a person is to developing symptoms, the more important it will be to use nicotinic acid, since it works more effectively than the amide. The amide dose may be small at first and gradually increase until 3–6 grams per day are being taken.

The optimum dose for vitamin B-3 is that quantity which is most effective in eliminating symptoms and has minimal or no side effects. This dose is maintained for life, but it may vary up or down. Each person must become skilled in determining what is the best dosage for himself.

Because water soluble vitamins such as niacin are excreted rapidly, it is best to divide the daily dosage into at least three doses. Ideally, you might take a much smaller quantity every hour, but this is not often practical. The controlled time release vitamin preparations drop vitamin B-3 into the body over an eight to twenty-four hour period to reproduce more accurately the slow rate of release of nutrients during the digestion of food. Also, the slow release tablet minimizes side effects, unless there is an allergy to the material used in binding the slow release granules.

Ascorbic Acid (Vitamin C)

Ascorbic acid must be listed as an antisenility vitamin, for it has the following properties which make it particularly valuable for elderly people:

1. *Vitamin C maintains the integrity of collagen.* Collagen is a major constituent of skin, one of the largest organs of the body, of bone and of many other organs. Its anticancer properties derive from this constituency in that healthy collagen tissue may resist the invasion of cancer cells better.

2. *Vitamin C increases resistance of the body against cancer.* For example, it prevents recurrences of cancer of the urinary bladder, against invasion by viruses and bacteria and reduces the ravages of allergic reactions.

Dr. B. V. Siegel (1975) found that ascorbic acid stimulated cells to increase production of interferon threefold. Interferon increases the ability of cells to resist penetration by viruses. In large doses, ascorbic acid has most valuable antiviral therapeutic properties. It reduces allergic reactions because it neutralizes histamine released into the blood.[3]

3. *Vitamin C is a valuable laxative.* Constipation is one of the difficulties faced by elderly people. The main reason is

lack of fiber, but a few elderly patients even on high fiber diets were constipated until placed upon optimum doses of ascorbic acid. It is much more beneficial than laxatives and is safe. Constipation can be especially damaging, not only for the mechanical reasons described under the Saccharine Disease, but because it decreases absorption of nutrients from the gut.

4. *Vitamin C prevents and reverses the effects of atherosclerosis when used for a long time.* Perhaps it does so by strengthening the collagen in the arterial walls.

The average healthy person will require 1–3 grams of vitamin C per day to remain healthy and a lot more when ill. Elderly people require triple this dose, and we recommend the dosage which just falls short of producing diarrhea. To find that dosage, increase the milligram intake until some diarrhea develops. Then reduce the dose a little.

Pantothenic Acid

Pantothenic acid was discovered by Roger Williams over thirty years ago, but it has been ignored almost as long. Prof. Williams reasoned it might have antiaging properties. He treated mice with this vitamin on top of a nutritious diet and found they lived 653 days when the control mice lived 550 days. In human terms, this would be equivalent to an increase in lifespan from seventy-five to eighty-nine years.

Pantothenic acid is required for normal functioning of the nervous system. In animals, severe deficiency leads to nerve degeneration. It also maintains the integrity of the immune system. Deficiency decreases the production of antibodies. It reinforces our defenses against stress by supporting the adrenal glands. Arthritics are also benefited. Dr. E. C. Bartin-Wright and W. A. Elliott, in the Rheumatic Clinic at St. Alfeges Hospital, London, tested 160 arthritics and found the blood level of pantothenic acid was 69 MCG per 100 ml of blood, only one-fourth to one-half that of normal controls. Giving arthritics pantothenic acid was beneficial.

It is prudent to take pantothenic acid as an antisenility nutrient at a dosage of 250 to 750 mg per day.

Tocopherol (Vitamin E)

There are eight vitamin E isomers in nature. D-alpha tocopherol is the most active biologically. Synthetic vitamin E is a racemic mixture including fractions not as active. Vitamin E is a powerful antioxidant by combining with free radicals or small highly active molecules.

Once life switched from anaerobic to aerobic respiration, it had to solve a major problem: how to prevent being oxidized (burned) by the oxygen in which it was immersed. This it did by developing antioxidants. When an apple or a potato turns brown when cut, this is oxidation. Oxidation must not be allowed to occur in the body. Plants develop antioxidants such as vitamin E. Animal tissue must also be protected, and it uses vitamin E as well as vitamin C and glutathione. Probably an accurate listing of all antioxidants is not yet available. Another antioxidant may be alpha tocopherylquinone, the main oxidation product of alpha tocopherol.

The amount of vitamin E required is not agreed upon because there is no clear relationship between vitamin E deficiency and disease in man. In animals, deficiency of vitamin E causes severe, often irreversible pathology. In one study on adult men, a diet containing only 5 IU per day showed a marked increase in the rate of destruction of red blood cells after six years. Yet, the daily recommended amount has been lowered from 30 to 15 IU per day. One reason for lowering this estimate was that dietitians were having difficulty in devising a diet which would provide more than 15 IU per day. Horwitt (1976) disagrees with this decision.[4]

We believe that even if 30 IU is adequate to protect us from increased wastage of red blood cells, it is altogether too low for optimum health. Several theories of aging invoke excessive oxidation. It is prudent to assume there is some validity to these ideas and to try and reverse these changes by large amounts of vitamin E. Thus Horwitt referred to a study where rats fed vitamin E equivalent to an average American diet suffered severe lung damage when exposed to 0.1 ppm ozone for seven days. Rats given six times as much vitamin E were not damaged.

Orthomolecular physicians have been using dosages of 400 IU and upward following the pioneering work of Evan Shute, M.D., and Wilfrid Shute, M.D. These dosages have been severely criticized by many as being unnecessary and even dangerous. The clinical trials of vitamin E as a treatment for coronary disease designed to refute the Shutes' work around 1950 used too little vitamin E for short periods of time. Horwitt points out that it takes a long time to saturate the tissues with vitamin E. He refers to studies which show that E prolonged blood clotting time.

Vitamin E is the last of the true antisenility vitamins we'll be discussing at length. The best dose ranges from 800 IU (International Units) to 1600 IU per day. This dose can be used immediately or arrived at slowly. We have already described its roles as an antioxidant or antisenility factor.

Many physicians appear to think that vitamin E is no better than placebo. The best evidence against this arises from diseases for which there is no treatment such as Huntington's chorea. The literature does not reveal that a single patient has ever been cured by having the illness halted and reversed. There are a small number of research papers which continue to report lists of treatments which have failed, but I have seen the condition respond to vitamin E.

Huntington's chorea is an inherited disease which appears in about 50 percent of the children of a parent with this disease. The progress of the disease is steadily downhill with a few plateaus, and there have been no recoveries. It is also very rare; so rare that I had not seen one case from 1945 when I became a medical student, until my first patient appeared about four years ago.

This patient had been ill twenty years and his father had died psychotic in a mental hospital, as had his father's brother. There were five sons with two having chronic Huntington's chorea and residing in nursing homes, hopelessly incapacitated and psychotic. One has died since then.

My patient was the third son in his family to come down with the disease. His weight had gone to 130 pounds from his normal 165 pounds. This was due to his loss of muscle mass. He was physically and mentally ill, and his mind was beginning to change. The young man was too suspicious, and at the same time indifferent or inappropriately euphoric. He walked with a limp, was so weak he could not raise his arms over his shoulders and the need to dress, eat and care for his personal needs required all his energy with none left for anything else.

He was started on a comprehensive program of ascorbic acid and water-soluble B-vitamins and after six months, he appeared to be stronger. In fact, he reported he was able to work in his garden and could do some repairs on his roof, but he had lost another five pounds. This was a very ominous sign since it indicated the disease was still progressing and muscle tissue was being wasted. At this time, I concluded he was really no better.

I then started him on vitamin E, 800 IU per day. I was aware of the use of vitamin E by veterinarian surgeons for treating muscular dystrophies. One month later, my patient's weight remained steady; after another month, he had gained four pounds, within four months, he weighed 137 pounds that was not fat. The man's muscles were rapidly regenerating and when last seen eight months ago, he had been nearly well for over two years. His weight has remained about 135. His wife stated the only sign of any residual disability occurred when he was very tense and walked with a slight limp.

Huntington's chorea is a cerebral degenerative disease which mimics the worst aspects of senility. Vitamin E was an important factor in this case, and if it can be so effective in halting progress of such a serious disease as Huntington's chorea, there is no longer any basis for the belief it is an inert substance. This is the first case of the condition recorded where the disease has been brought under control.

Of course, vitamin E is one of the most valuable substances in controlling cardiovascular disease.

Other Vitamins

Other vitamins non-specific as antisenility factors will be needed if there are special indications. These include vitamin A if there are special problems with the skin or eyes; vitamin D-3 if there are problems with calcium metabolism; vitamin K if bruises develop too easily; and folic acid and vitamin B 12 if blood levels are low. Any one of these may be required in optimum doses.

Pyridoxine (vitamin B-6) is such an important nutrient it seems only prudent to use it as a supplement. It is involved in a large number of vital metabolic reactions. Up to 500 mg per day should be taken and more if there are clinical indications of pyridoxine dependency.

References for Chapter Seven

1. Bowerman, W.M. A review of Korsakoff's three papers on the syndrome which bears his name. Personal communication, 1978.

2. Centerwall, Brandon. Put thiamine in liquor. *The New York Times*, February 12, 1979.

3. Siegel, B.V. Enhancement of interferon production by poly (RI). poly (RC) in mouse cell cultures by ascorbic acid. *Nature* 254:531-532, 1975.

4. Horwitt, M.K. Vitamin E: a re-examination. *American Journal of Clinical Nutrition* 29:569-578, 1976.

DIETARY MINERALS
AND OTHER ASPECTS
OF GOOD NUTRITION

A surprising variant of the proposition that you are what you eat is being explored as a promising strategy for dealing with some forms of memory impairment, which is among the most distressing, difficult and common afflictions of old age. The memory problems experienced by some elderly people probably have less to do with specific diseases of aging than with the combined effects of poor nutrition, loneliness and social deprivation.
—Harold M. Schmeck, Jr., *The New York Times*, January 9, 1979

The Long Life You Enjoy from Eating Minerals

"CHARLIE SMITH and the Fritter Tree," was televised October 9, 1978, by the Public Broadcasting Service. It showed the life story of 136-year-old Charlie Smith, and Mr. Smith was around to see it.[1]

The film traced his life from the time he was taken from Africa when he was twelve years old and was put aboard a slave ship for bondage in Texas, until his freedom in 1863, because of the Emancipation Proclamation. It depicted him as a cowhand, an outlaw who rode with Jesse James, a bounty hunter, a fruit picker and finally a grand old story-teller.

Most all of his life, Charlie Smith rode the range on his

153

horse as a cowpoke. He hustled those longhorn steers and ate their trail dust pushing them on to market. The secret of the cowboy's longevity is probably the very dust he found distasteful. There are many minerals in it.

Of the six nutrients that our bodies need, minerals, vitamins, water, protein, carbohydrates and fats, dietary minerals have the power to keep us young and rejuvenate our bodies. Minerals are actively engaged in strengthening our nervous system, growing new hair, normalizing the heartbeat, providing a powerhouse of energy, improving our thinking power, overcoming fatigue, building a dynamic memory, and sparking our other metabolic processes.

Mineral imbalance will alter one's disposition. In a mineral deficient person, you'll see signs of forgetfulness, easy fatigue, lack of incentive, lack-luster skin and hair, grouchiness, short temper, nervous tension, defeatism, depression, revengefulness, resignation to failure in life, and suicidal tendencies. In fact, if anyone has a shortage of just one mineral, he can expect that his system will begin to weaken and lose its efficiency with disease eventually setting in.

There are two categories of dietary minerals: major minerals and trace minerals. Major minerals are needed in large amounts by the body. Trace minerals get their name from the fact that they are found in very minute amounts in the body and may be toxic to us in larger quantities.

Taking minerals in regulated amounts in foods rich in minerals or as mineral supplements will ensure a long life. They have the ability to regulate the flow of bodily fluids. The delicate internal water balance needed for all mental and physical processes through osmosis is necessary for good health. It brings the cells oxygen and nutrition and empties them of wastes. The minerals draw these substances into and out of our cells by the law of mass action in which areas with a heavier concentration of minerals will always draw water from the areas with a lighter concentration of minerals. In this way, concentration is equalized between the fluids in the cells and the fluids without as an ongoing body process.

The bodily fluids, solutions of water and dissolved mineral salts, hold the cells in electrolyte balance. The mineral salts each generate a tiny electrical charge, either positive or negative. Each cell is similar to a minute electrical battery, with both positive and negative polarities receiving the electrolytic solution containing the essential chemicals and minerals it needs. Give the cells the minerals they need, and they will give you long life and good health.

Particular Dietary Minerals Required by the Elderly

We are not aware of studies which link any particular mineral to senility, but certain ones are more necessary for the elderly. Rather than acquire one's supply of minerals from supplementation, we recommend your getting them from eating an abundance of fresh fruits and vegetables, nuts and grains. Fresh foods contain many more minerals in a natural balance than processed foods. If fresh foods are not available, homeopathic cell salts may be purchased in a health food store. They are also available as a combination tablet containing twelve mineral salts.

Or, you may wish to take chelated minerals. *A chelated mineral atom* is one that is surrounded or enclosed by a larger protein molecule. The chelation process changes the positive ionic (electrolyte) charge to a negative ionic charge, making it more acceptable through the villi of the intestines into the blood stream, where it can be used easily and efficiently by the body.

Of the fourteen major and trace minerals necessary for life, three in particular are recommended to reduce the effects of aging. They are calcium, magnesium, and zinc.

Calcium is the most abundant mineral in the body, and the bones and teeth hold 99 percent of it. Osteoporosis and periodontal disease, both manifestations of calcium deficiency, are common in the elderly. Osteoporosis may appear as early as age twenty-five, but it is more common in women toward the end of life. In the Sudan where calcium intake may exceed 2 grams per day, periodontal disease and spinal bone disease are rare.

The recommended dosage of calcium supplement is 1 gram a day, but we think twice as much for an older person would be better. Herta Spencer, M.D., of the Veterans Administration Hospital in Hines, Illinois, suggests 1200 mg per day. The U.S. Government's recommended daily allowance (RDA) is only 800 mg a day. Dr. Spencer also found that aluminum antacids, even in small doses, can damage bones by the loss of both calcium and magnesium, which could lead to osteomalacia.

Magnesium, an essential mineral, occurs in the body in appreciable quantities. The adult body contains about 25 grams, 70 percent of which is combined with calcium and phosphorus in the bone salt complex. Magnesium aids in the absorption of calcium. It is one of four cations that must be in balance in extracellular fluids so that the transmission of nerve impulses and the subsequent muscle contraction can be regulated.

The National Research Council of the United States recommends a daily magnesium intake of 350 mg for the adult male and 300 mg for the adult female. Since the average American diet barely provides anything near even this inadequate RDA, we believe this dosage should be tripled. Otherwise, the deficiency of magnesium will show up as symptoms of senility including mental confusion, disorientation, apprehensiveness, muscle twitching, tremors, and blood vessel clots.

Zinc, a trace metal, is extremely important in the synthesis of RNA, DNA and protein, and is essential in maintaining an adequate blood level of vitamin A. There are seventy known enzymes that contain zinc. One of these breaks down a molecule called superoxide, which accumulates in sites of inflammation of rheumatoid arthritis. In one study, sixteen elderly patients were able to take 220 mg of zinc sulphate three times a day with minimal side effects. If any diarrhea occurs, lower doses, or a different salt such as zinc gluconate may be used.

Zinc salts are water soluble and thus easily lost from the body. In contrast to iron, which can be conserved, zinc has to be taken every day as do vitamins. We consider zinc an important antisenility mineral because a deficiency in elderly people can cause a confusional state, which may be mistaken as senility. Lack of zinc causes a disorder of taste and smell resulting in reduced food consumption. In men, zinc in adequate doses decreases the probability of prostate enlargement. The average zinc content of a mixed diet is between 10 and 15 mg. Since this mineral is relatively nontoxic and such an important mineral, we recommend taking 45 mg per day by the older person.

Some people will require a dosage range of 30 mg to 100 mg per day of zinc gluconate or 200 to 660 mg of zinc sulphate. The higher doses are necessary for special needs such as a deficiency in taste or smell, or chalky white areas on the nails or prostate trouble.

The Nutrient Content of Foods

As we stated, it is best to acquire all of the daily allotment of nutrients you need from the nutritional quality of foods eaten. We have, therefore, supplied a listing by courtesy of Dan Black, President of Nutrilab, Inc., 22455 Maple Court, Suite 305, Hayward, California 99451. It shows the vitamin and mineral content of many foods for you to tailor your eating to specific dietary needs. Use the listing to identify foods that are good sources for the particular vitamin or mineral you are interested in.

While the values given in these lists can be useful in comparing their content in foods, absolute values for food nutrients will be variable depending on such factors as the condition of the soil where the food was grown, amount of processing or refining, and method of preparation.

The quantity of each food on the lists has been standardized to 100 grams, rather than listing them in common measurements. This provides a more appropriate comparison between relative amounts of nutrients in foods and allows them to be ranked from highest to lowest. Remember, not all foods are consumed in 100 gram quantities as they may be highly concentrated, such as kelp, dulse, wheat germ and brewer's yeast. These foods often appear at the top of the list indicating them as concentrated nutritional sources. To give an idea of what 100 grams of a food represents in common measurements, the following conversions may be useful:

Approximate Equivalents

1 teaspoon fluid	=	About 5 grams
1 teaspoon dry	=	About 4 grams
1 cup milk, yogurt	=	245 grams
1 cup leafy vegetable	=	90 grams
1 cup root vegetable	=	135 grams
1 cup nuts, seeds	=	140 grams
1 cup sliced fruit	=	150 grams
1 cup cereal grain, uncooked	=	200 grams
1 tablespoon cooking oil	=	14 grams
1 tablespoon honey, molasses	=	20 grams

Carotene—vitamin A

IU per 100 grams edible portion (100 grams = 3½ oz.)

50,500	Liver, lamb	10,900	Apricots, dried
43,900	Liver, beef	9,300	Collard leaves
22,500	Liver, calf	8,900	Kale
21,600	Peppers, red chili	8,800	Sweet potatoes
14,000	Dandelion greens	8,500	Parsley
12,100	Liver, chicken	8,100	Spinach
11,000	Carrots	7,600	Turnip greens

7,000	Mustard greens	1,580	Swordfish
6,500	Swiss chard	1,540	Cream, whipping
6,100	Beet greens	1,330	Peaches
5,800	Chives	1,200	Acorn squash
5,700	Butternut squash	1,180	Eggs
4,900	Watercress	1,080	Chicken
4,800	Mangos	1,000	Cherries, sour red
4,450	Peppers, sweet red	970	Butterhead lettuce
4,300	Hubbard squash	900	Asparagus
3,400	Cantaloupe	900	Tomatoes, ripe
3,300	Butter	770	Peppers, green chili
3,300	Endive	690	Kidneys
2,700	Apricots	640	Green peas
2,500	Broccoli spears	600	Green beans
2,260	Whitefish	600	Elderberries
2,000	Green onions	590	Watermelon
1,900	Romaine lettuce	580	Rutabagas
1,750	Papayas	550	Brussels sprouts
1,650	Nectarines	520	Okra
1,600	Prunes	510	Yellow cornmeal
1,600	Pumpkin	460	Yellow squash

Vitamin A from animal source foods occurs mostly as active, preformed vitamin A (retinol) while that from vegetable source foods occurs as pro-vitamin A (beta-carotene and other carotenoids) which must be converted to active vitamin A by the body to be utilized. The efficiency of conversion varies among individuals; however, beta-carotene is converted more efficiently than other carotenoids. Green and deep yellow vegetables as well as deep yellow fruits are highest in beta-carotene.

Tocopherol—vitamin E

IU per 100 grams edible portion (100 grams = 3½ oz.)

216	Wheat germ oil	45	Sesame oil
90	Sunflower seeds	34	Peanut oil
88	Sunflower seed oil	29	Corn oil
72	Safflower oil	22	Wheat germ
48	Almonds	18	Peanuts

18	Olive oil	2.2	Rye bread, dark
14	Soybean oil	1.9	Pecans
13	Peanuts, roasted	1.9	Wheat germ
11	Peanut butter	1.9	Rye & wheat crackers
3.6	Butter	1.4	Whole wheat bread
3.2	Spinach	1.0	Carrots
3.0	Oatmeal	.99	Peas
3.0	Bran	.92	Walnuts
2.9	Asparagus	.88	Bananas
2.5	Salmon	.83	Eggs
2.5	Brown rice	.72	Tomatoes
2.3	Rye, whole	.29	Lamb

Calciferol (synthetic)—vitamin D

IU per 100 grams edible portion (100 grams = 3½ oz.)

500	Sardines, canned	50	Liver
350	Salmon	50	Eggs
250	Tuna	40	Milk, fortified
150	Shrimp	40	Mushrooms
90	Butter	30	Natural cheeses
90	Sunflower seeds		

Vitamin K

Micrograms (mcg) per 100 grams edible portion
(100 grams = 3½ oz.)

650	Turnip greens	17	Whole wheat
200	Broccoli	14	Green beans
129	Lettuce	11	Pork
125	Cabbage	11	Eggs
92	Beef liver	10	Corn oil
89	Spinach	8	Peaches
57	Watercress	7	Beef
57	Asparagus	7	Chicken liver
35	Cheese	6	Raisins
30	Butter	5	Tomato
25	Pork liver	3	Milk
20	Oats	3	Potato
19	Green peas		

Thiamine—vitamin B-1

Milligrams (mg) per 100 grams edible portion
(100 grams = 3½ oz.)

15.61	Yeast, brewer's	.45	Heart, lamb
14.01	Yeast, torula	.45	Wild rice
2.01	Wheat germ	.43	Cashews
1.96	Sunflower seeds	.43	Rye, whole-grain
1.84	Rice polishings	.40	Liver, lamb
1.28	Pine nuts	.40	Lobster
1.14	Peanuts, with skins	.38	Mung beans
1.10	Soybeans, dry	.38	Cornmeal,
1.05	Cowpeas, dry		whole-ground
.98	Peanuts, without skins	.37	Lentils
.96	Brazil nuts	.36	Kidneys, beef
.93	Pork, lean	.35	Green peas
.86	Pecans	.34	Macadamia nuts
.85	Soybean flour	.34	Brown rice
.84	Beans, pinto & red	.33	Walnuts
.74	Split peas	.31	Garbanzos
.73	Millet	.30	Liver, pork
.72	Wheat bran	.25	Garlic, cloves
.67	Pistachio nuts	.25	Liver, beef
.65	Navy beans	.24	Almonds
.63	Heart, veal	.24	Lima beans, fresh
.60	Buckwheat	.24	Pumpkin & squash
.60	Oatmeal		seeds
.55	Whole wheat flour	.23	Brains, all kinds
.55	Whole wheat	.23	Chestnuts, fresh
.51	Kidneys, lamb	.23	Soybean sprouts
.48	Lima beans, dry	.22	Peppers, red chili
.46	Hazelnuts	.18	Sesame seeds,
			hulled

Riboflavin—vitamin B-2

Milligrams (mg) per 100 grams edible portion
(100 grams = 3½ oz.)

5.06	Yeast, torula	3.28	Liver, lamb
4.28	Yeast, brewer's	3.26	Liver, beef

3.03	Liver, pork	.26	Kale
2.72	Liver, calf	.26	Parsley
2.55	Kidneys, beef	.25	Cashews
2.49	Liver, chicken	.25	Rice bran
2.42	Kidneys, lamb	.25	Veal
1.36	Chicken giblets	.24	Lamb, lean
1.05	Heart, veal	.23	Broccoli
.92	Almonds	.23	Chicken, flesh & skin
.88	Heart, beef		
.74	Heart, lamb	.23	Pine nuts
.68	Wheat germ	.23	Salmon
.63	Wild rice	.23	Sunflower seeds
.46	Mushrooms	.22	Navy beans
.44	Egg yolks	.22	Beet & mustard greens
.38	Millet		
.36	Peppers, hot red	.22	Lentils
.35	Soy flour	.22	Pork, lean
.35	Wheat bran	.22	Prunes
.33	Mackerel	.22	Rye, whole grain
.31	Collards	.21	Mung beans
.31	Soybeans, dry	.21	Beans, pinto & red
.30	Eggs	.21	Blackeye peas
.29	Split peas	.21	Okra
.29	Tongue, beef	.13	Sesame seeds, hulled
.26	Brains, all kinds		

Niacin—vitamin B-3

Milligrams (mg) per 100 grams edible portion
(100 grams = 3½ oz.)

44.4	Yeast, torula	11.4	Liver, calf
37.9	Yeast, brewer's	11.3	Turkey, light meat
29.8	Rice bran	10.8	Liver, chicken
28.2	Rice polishings	10.7	Chicken, light meat
21.0	Wheat bran	8.4	Trout
17.2	Peanuts, with skins	8.3	Halibut
16.9	Liver, lamb	8.2	Mackerel
16.4	Liver, pork	8.1	Heart, veal
15.8	Peanuts, without skins	8.0	Chicken, flesh only
13.6	Liver, beef	8.0	Swordfish

8.0	Turkey, flesh only	4.7	Brown rice
7.7	Goose, flesh only	4.5	Pine nuts
7.5	Heart, beef	4.4	Buckwheat, whole-grain
7.2	Salmon		
6.4	Veal	4.4	Peppers, red chili
6.4	Kidneys, beef	4.4	Whole wheat grain
6.2	Wild rice	4.3	Whole wheat flour
6.1	Chicken giblets	4.2	Mushrooms
5.7	Lamb, lean	4.2	Wheat germ
5.6	Chicken, flesh & skin	3.7	Barley
		3.6	Herring
5.4	Sesame seeds	3.5	Almonds
5.4	Sunflower seeds	3.5	Shrimp
5.1	Beef, lean	3.0	Haddock
5.0	Pork, lean	3.0	Split peas

Pantothenic acid—a B vitamin

Milligrams (mg) per 100 grams edible portion
(100 grams = 3½ oz.)

12.0	Yeast, brewer's	1.4	Lentils
11.0	Yeast, torula	1.3	Rye flour, whole
8.0	Liver, calf	1.3	Cashews
6.0	Liver, chicken	1.3	Salmon, flesh
3.9	Kidneys, beef	1.2	Camembert cheese
2.8	Peanuts	1.2	Garbanzos
2.6	Brains, all kinds	1.2	Wheat germ, toasted
2.6	Heart	1.2	Broccoli
2.2	Mushrooms	1.1	Hazelnuts
2.0	Soybean flour	1.1	Turkey, dark meat
2.0	Split peas	1.1	Brown rice
2.0	Tongue, beef	1.1	Wheat flour, whole
1.9	Perch	1.1	Sardines
1.8	Blue cheese	1.1	Peppers, red chili
1.7	Pecans	1.1	Avocados
1.7	Soybeans	1.1	Veal, lean
1.6	Eggs	1.0	Blackeye peas, dry
1.5	Lobster	1.0	Wild rice
1.5	Oatmeal, dry	1.0	Cauliflower
1.4	Buckwheat flour	1.0	Chicken, dark meat
1.4	Sunflower seeds	1.0	Kale

Pyridoxine—vitamin B-6

Milligrams (mg) per 100 grams edible portion
(100 grams = 3½ oz.)

3.00	Yeast, torula	.43	Kidneys, beef
2.50	Yeast, brewer's	.42	Avocados
1.25	Sunflower seeds	.41	Kidneys, veal
1.15	Wheat germ, toasted	.34	Whole wheat flour
.90	Tuna, flesh	.33	Chestnuts, fresh
.84	Liver, beef	.30	Egg yolks
.81	Soybeans, dry	.30	Kale
.75	Liver, chicken	.30	Rye flour
.73	Walnuts	.28	Spinach
.70	Salmon, flesh	.26	Turnip greens
.69	Trout, flesh	.26	Peppers, sweet
.67	Liver, calf	.25	Heart, beef
.66	Mackerel, flesh	.25	Potatoes
.65	Liver, pork	.24	Prunes
.63	Soybean flour	.24	Raisins
.60	Lentils, dry	.24	Sardines
.58	Lima beans, dry	.24	Brussels sprouts
.58	Buckwheat flour	.23	Elderberries
.56	Blackeye peas, dry	.23	Perch, flesh
.56	Navy beans, dry	.22	Cod, flesh
.55	Brown rice	.22	Barley
.54	Hazelnuts	.22	Cheese, camembert
.54	Garbanzos, dry	.22	Sweet potatoes
.53	Pinto beans, dry	.21	Cauliflower
.51	Bananas	.20	Popcorn, popped
.45	Pork, lean	.20	Red cabbage
.44	Albacore, flesh	.20	Leeks
.43	Beef, lean	.20	Molasses
.43	Halibut, flesh		

Folic acid—a B vitamin

Micrograms (mcg) per 100 grams edible portion
(100 grams = 3½ oz.)

2022	Brewer's yeast	430	Rice germ
440	Blackeye peas	425	Soy flour

305	Wheat germ	53	Broccoli
295	Liver, beef	50	Barley
275	Liver, lamb	50	Split peas
220	Liver, pork	49	Whole wheat
225	Soybeans		cereal
195	Bran	49	Brussels sprouts
180	Kidney beans	45	Almonds
145	Mung beans	38	Whole wheat flour
130	Lima beans	33	Oatmeal
125	Navy beans	32	Cabbage
125	Garbanzos	32	Dried figs
110	Asparagus	30	Avocado
105	Lentils	28	Green beans
77	Walnuts	28	Corn
75	Spinach, fresh	28	Coconut, fresh
70	Kale	27	Pecans
65	Filbert nuts	25	Mushrooms
60	Beet & mustard greens	25	Dates
57	Textured vegetable	14	Blackberries
	protein	7	Ground beef
56	Peanuts, roasted	5	Orange
56	Peanut butter		

Cobalamin—vitamin B-12

Micrograms (mcg) per 100 grams edible portion
(100 grams = 3½ oz.)

104	Liver, lamb	4.0	Salmon, flesh
98	Clams	3.0	Tuna, flesh
80	Liver, beef	2.1	Lamb
63	Kidneys, lamb	2.1	Sweetbreads (thymus)
60	Liver, calf	2.0	Eggs
31	Kidneys, beef	2.0	Whey, dried
25	Liver, chicken	1.8	Beef, lean
18	Oysters	1.8	Edam cheese
17	Sardines	1.8	Swiss cheese
11	Heart, beef	1.6	Brie cheese
6	Egg yolks	1.6	Gruyere cheese
5.2	Heart, lamb	1.4	Blue cheese
5.0	Trout	1.3	Haddock, flesh
4.0	Brains, all kinds	1.2	Flounder, flesh

1.2	Scallops	1.0	Halibut
1.0	Cheddar cheese	1.0	Perch, fillets
1.0	Cottage cheese	1.0	Swordfish, flesh
1.0	Mozzarella cheese		

Biotin—a B vitamin

Micrograms (mcg) per 100 grams edible portion
(100 grams = 3½ oz.)

200	Brewer's yeast	24	Sardines, canned
127	Liver, lamb	22	Whole egg
100	Liver, pork	21	Blackeye peas
96	Liver, beef	18	Split peas
70	Soy flour	18	Almonds
61	Soybeans	17	Cauliflower
60	Rice bran	16	Mushrooms
58	Rice germ	16	Whole wheat cereal
57	Rice polishings	15	Salmon, canned
52	Egg yolk	15	Textured vegetable
39	Peanut butter		protein
37	Walnuts	14	Bran
34	Peanuts, roasted	13	Lentils
31	Barley	12	Brown rice
27	Pecans	10	Chicken
24	Oatmeal		

Choline—a B vitamin

Milligrams (mg) per 100 grams edible portion
(100 grams = 3½ oz.)

2200	Lecithin	223	Lentils
1490	Egg yolk	201	Split peas
550	Liver	170	Rice bran
504	Whole egg	162	Peanuts, roasted
406	Wheat germ	156	Oatmeal
340	Soybeans	145	Peanut butter
300	Rice germ	143	Bran
257	Blackeye peas	139	Barley
245	Garbanzo beans	122	Ham
240	Brewer's yeast	112	Brown rice

104	Veal	42	Green beans
102	Rice polishings	29	Potatoes
94	Whole wheat cereal	23	Cabbage
86	Molasses	22	Spinach
77	Pork	20.5	Textured vegetable
75	Beef		protein
75	Green peas	15	Milk
66	Sweet potatoes	12	Orange juice
48	Cheddar cheese	5	Butter

Inositol—a B vitamin

Milligrams (mg) per 100 grams edible portion
(100 grams = 3½ oz.)

2200	Lecithin	150	Grapefruit
770	Wheat germ	130	Lentils
500	Navy beans	120	Raisins
460	Rice bran	120	Cantaloupe
454	Rice polishings	119	Brown rice
390	Cooked barley	117	Orange juice
370	Rice germ	110	Whole wheat flour
370	Whole wheat	96	Peaches
270	Brewer's yeast	95	Cabbage
270	Oatmeal	95	Cauliflower
240	Blackeye peas	88	Onion
240	Garbanzo beans	67	Whole wheat bread
210	Orange	66	Sweet potatoes
205	Soy flour	64	Watermelon
200	Soybeans	60	Strawberries
180	Peanuts, roasted	55	Lettuce
180	Peanut butter	51	Beef liver
170	Lima beans	46	Tomato
162	Green peas	33	Egg
150	Molasses	13	Milk
150	Split peas	11	Beef, round

Ascorbic acid—vitamin C

Milligrams (mg) per 100 grams edible portion
(100 grams = 3½ oz.)

| 1300 | Acerola | 242 | Guavas |
| 369 | Peppers, red chili | 204 | Peppers, red sweet |

186	Kale leaves	33	Asparagus
172	Parsley	33	Cantaloupes
152	Collard leaves	32	Swiss chard
139	Turnip greens	32	Green onions
128	Peppers, green sweet	31	Liver, beef
113	Broccoli	31	Okra
102	Brussels sprouts	31	Tangerines
97	Mustard greens	30	New Zealand
79	Watercress		spinach
78	Cauliflower	30	Oysters
66	Persimmons	29	Lima beans, young
61	Cabbage, red	29	Blackeye peas
59	Strawberries	29	Soybeans
56	Papayas	27	Green peas
51	Spinach	26	Radishes
50	Oranges and juice	25	Raspberries
47	Cabbage	25	Chinese cabbage
46	Lemon juice	25	Yellow summer
38	Grapefruit and juice		squash
36	Elderberries	24	Loganberries
36	Liver, calf	23	Honeydew melon
36	Turnips	23	Tomatoes
35	Mangos	23	Liver, pork

Amygdalin—vitamin B-17

HIGH—Above 500 milligrams (mg) per
100 grams edible portion

Wild blackberry
Elderberry
Apple seeds
Apricot seeds
Cherry seeds
Nectarine seeds
Peach seed
Pear seed

Plum seed
Prune seed
Fava beans
Mung beans
Bitter almond
Macadamia nuts
Bamboo sprouts
Alfalfa leaves

MEDIUM—Above 100 milligrams (mg) per 100 grams edible portion

Boysenberry
Currant
Gooseberry
Huckleberry
Loganberry
Mulberry
Quince
Raspberry
Alfalfa sprouts
Buckwheat

Flax seed
Millet
Squash-seed
Mung bean sprouts
Garbanzo beans
Blackeye peas
Kidney beans
Lentils
Lima beans

LOW—Below 100 milligrams (mg) per 100 grams edible portion

Commercial blackberry
Cranberry
Black beans
Green peas
Lima beans

Sweet potatoes, yams
Cashews
Beet tops
Spinach
Watercress

Para-aminobenzoic acid (PABA)—a B vitamin

Mushrooms
Liver
Bran
Cabbage
Sunflower seeds

Wheat germ
Oats
Spinach
Whole milk
Eggs

Pangamic acid—vitamin B-15

Apricot kernels
Yeast
Liver
Rice bran
Corn grits
Wheat germ

Sunflower seeds
Pumpkin seeds
Oat grits
Wheat bran
Whole grain cereals

Bioflavonoids—vitamin P

Grapes	Grapefruit
Rose hips	Cabbage
Prunes	Apricots
Orange	Peppers
Lemon juice	Papaya
Cherries	Cantaloupe
Black currant	Tomato
Plums	Broccoli
Parsley	Blackberry

As food sources with appreciable quantities of the above nutrients are few, a listing of the best sources of these nutrients is given instead of showing relative nutrient amounts.

Calcium

Milligrams (mg) per 100 grams edible portion
(100 grams = 3½ oz.)

1093	Kelp	120	Sunflower seeds
925	Swiss cheese	120	Yogurt
750	Cheddar cheese	119	Beet greens
352	Carob flour	119	Wheat bran
296	Dulse	118	Whole milk
250	Collard leaves	114	Buckwheat, raw
246	Turnip greens	110	Sesame seeds, hulled
245	Barbados molasses	106	Ripe olives
234	Almonds	103	Broccoli
210	Brewer's yeast	99	English walnut
203	Parsley	94	Cottage cheese
200	Corn tortillas (lime added)	93	Spinach
		73	Soybeans, cooked
187	Dandelion greens	73	Pecans
186	Brazil nuts	72	Wheat germ
151	Watercress	69	Peanuts
129	Goat milk	68	Miso
128	Tofu	68	Romaine lettuce
126	Dried figs	67	Dried apricots
121	Buttermilk	66	Rutabaga

62	Raisins	26	Fresh green peas
60	Black currant	25	Cauliflower
59	Dates	25	Lentils, cooked
56	Green snap beans	22	Sweet cherry
51	Globe artichokes	22	Asparagus
51	Dried prunes	22	Winter squash
51	Pumpkin and	21	Strawberry
	squash seeds	20	Millet
50	Cooked dry beans	19	Mung bean sprouts
49	Common cabbage	17	Pineapple
48	Soybean sprouts	16	Grapes
46	Hard winter wheat	16	Beets
41	Orange	14	Cantaloupe
39	Celery	14	Jerusalem arti-
38	Cashews		choke
38	Rye grain	13	Tomato
37	Carrot	12	Eggplant
34	Barley	12	Chicken
32	Sweet potato	11	Orange juice
32	Brown rice	10	Avocado
29	Garlic	10	Beef
28	Summer squash	8	Banana
27	Onion	7	Apple
26	Lemon	3	Sweet corn

Magnesium

Milligrams (mg) per 100 grams edible portion
(100 grams = 3½ oz.)

760	Kelp	175	Peanuts
490	Wheat bran	162	Millet
336	Wheat germ	160	Wheat grain
270	Almonds	142	Pecan
267	Cashews	131	English walnut
258	Blackstrap molasses	115	Rye
231	Brewer's yeast	111	Tofu
229	Buckwheat	106	Beet greens
225	Brazil nut	90	Coconut meat, dry
220	Dulse	88	Soybeans, cooked
184	Filberts	88	Spinach

88	Brown rice	30	Blackberry
71	Dried figs	25	Beets
65	Swiss chard	24	Broccoli
62	Apricots, dried	24	Cauliflower
58	Dates	23	Carrot
57	Collard leaves	22	Celery
51	Shrimp	21	Beef
48	Sweet corn	20	Asparagus
45	Avocado	19	Chicken
45	Cheddar cheese	18	Green pepper
41	Parsley	17	Winter squash
40	Prunes, dried	16	Cantaloupe
38	Sunflower seeds	16	Eggplant
37	Common beans, cooked	14	Tomato
		13	Cabbage
37	Barley	13	Grapes
36	Dandelion greens	13	Milk
36	Garlic	13	Pineapple
35	Raisins	13	Mushroom
35	Fresh green peas	12	Onion
34	Potato with skin	11	Orange
34	Crab	11	Iceberg lettuce
33	Banana	9	Plum
31	Sweet potato	8	Apple

Phosphorus

Milligrams (mg) per 100 grams edible portion
(100 grams = 3½ oz.)

1753	Brewer's yeast	380	English walnut
1276	Wheat bran	376	Rye grain
1144	Pumpkin and squash seeds	373	Cashews
		352	Beef liver
1118	Wheat germ	338	Scallops
837	Sunflower seeds	311	Millet
693	Brazil nuts	290	Barley, pearled
592	Sesame seeds, hulled	289	Pecans
554	Soybeans, dried	267	Dulse
504	Almonds	240	Kelp
478	Cheddar cheese	239	Chicken
457	Pinto beans, dried	221	Brown rice
409	Peanuts	205	Eggs
400	Wheat	202	Garlic

175	Crab	44	Pumpkin
152	Cottage cheese	42	Avocado
150	Beef or lamb	40	Beet greens
119	Lentils, cooked	39	Swiss chard
116	Mushrooms	38	Winter squash
116	Fresh peas	36	Carrot
111	Sweet corn	36	Onions
101	Raisins	35	Red cabbage
93	Whole cow's milk	33	Beets
88	Globe artichoke	31	Radish
87	Yogurt	29	Summer squash
80	Brussels sprouts	28	Celery
79	Prunes, dried	27	Cucumber
78	Broccoli	27	Tomato
77	Figs, dried	26	Banana
69	Yams	26	Persimmon
67	Soybean sprouts	26	Eggplant
64	Mung bean sprouts	26	Lettuce
63	Dates	24	Nectarine
63	Parsley	22	Raspberry
62	Asparagus	20	Grapes
59	Bamboo shoots	20	Orange
56	Cauliflower	17	Olives
53	Potato with skin	16	Cantaloupe
51	Okra	10	Apple
51	Spinach	8	Pineapple
44	Green beans		

Sodium

Milligrams (mg) per 100 grams edible portion
(100 grams = 3½ oz.)

3007	Kelp	130	Buttermilk
2400	Green olives	126	Celery
1428	Dill pickles	122	Eggs
828	Ripe olives	110	Cod
747	Sauerkraut	71	Spinach
700	Cheddar cheese	70	Lamb
265	Scallops	65	Pork
229	Cottage cheese	64	Chicken
210	Lobster	60	Beef
147	Swiss chard	60	Beets
130	Beet greens	60	Sesame seeds

52	Watercress	19	White beans
50	Whole cow's milk	15	Broccoli
49	Turnip	15	Mushrooms
47	Carrot	13	Cauliflower
47	Yogurt	10	Onion
45	Parsley	10	Sweet potato
43	Artichoke	9	Brown rice
34	Dried figs	9	Lettuce
30	Lentils, dried	6	Cucumber
30	Sunflower seeds	5	Peanuts
27	Raisins	4	Avocado
26	Red cabbage	3	Tomato
19	Garlic	2	Eggplant
		2132	Salt, 1 tsp.
		1319	Soy sauce, 1 tbl.

The following foods contain large amounts of sodium chloride added during processing and should generally be avoided:

Canned or frozen vegetables	Luncheon meats
Cured, smoked, or canned meats	Salted nuts
Packaged spice mixes	Salted crackers
Bouillon cubes	Canned or packaged soups
Canned fish	Processed cheeses
Commercial peanut butter	Commercial salad dressings
Potato chips, corn chips, pretzels, etc.	Meat tenderizers

Potassium

Milligrams (mg) per 100 grams edible portion
(100 grams = 3½ oz.)

8060	Dulse	715	Brazil nuts
5273	Kelp	674	Peanuts
920	Sunflower seeds	648	Dates
827	Wheat germ	640	Figs, dried
773	Almonds	604	Avocado
763	Raisins	603	Pecans
727	Parsley	600	Yams

550	Swiss chard	244	Tomato
540	Soybeans, cooked	243	Sweet potato
529	Garlic	234	Papaya
470	Spinach	214	Eggplant
450	English walnut	213	Green pepper
430	Millet	208	Beets
416	Beans, cooked	202	Peach
414	Mushrooms	202	Summer squash
407	Potato with skin	200	Orange
382	Broccoli	199	Raspberries
370	Banana	191	Cherries
370	Meats	164	Strawberry
369	Winter squash	162	Grapefruit juice
366	Chicken	158	Grapes
341	Carrots	157	Onions
341	Celery	146	Pineapple
322	Radishes	144	Milk, whole
295	Cauliflower	141	Lemon juice
282	Watercress	130	Pear
278	Asparagus	129	Eggs
268	Red cabbage	110	Apple
264	Lettuce	100	Watermelon
251	Cantaloupe	70	Brown rice, cooked
249	Lentils, cooked		

Iron

Milligrams (mg) per 100 grams edible portion
(100 grams = 3½ oz.)

100.3	Kelp	3.9	Dried prunes
17.3	Brewer's yeast	3.8	Cashews
16.1	Blackstrap molasses	3.7	Lean beef
14.9	Wheat bran	3.5	Raisins
11.2	Pumpkin and squash	3.4	Jerusalem artichoke
	seeds	3.4	Brazil nuts
9.4	Wheat germ	3.3	Beet greens
8.8	Beef liver	3.2	Swiss chard
7.1	Sunflower seeds	3.1	Dandelion greens
6.8	Millet	3.1	English walnut
6.2	Parsley	3.0	Dates
6.1	Clams	2.9	Pork
4.7	Almonds	2.7	Cooked dry beans

2.4	Sesame seeds, hulled	0.8	Mushrooms
2.4	Pecans	0.7	Banana
2.3	Eggs	0.7	Beets
2.1	Lentils	0.7	Carrot
2.1	Peanuts	0.7	Eggplant
1.9	Lamb	0.7	Sweet potato
1.9	Tofu	0.6	Avocado
1.8	Green peas	0.6	Figs
1.6	Brown rice	0.6	Potato
1.6	Ripe olives	0.6	Corn
1.5	Chicken	0.5	Pineapple
1.3	Artichoke	0.5	Nectarine
1.3	Mung bean sprouts	0.5	Watermelon
1.2	Salmon	0.5	Winter squash
1.1	Broccoli	0.5	Brown rice, cooked
1.1	Currants	0.5	Tomato
1.1	Whole wheat bread	0.4	Orange
1.1	Cauliflower	0.4	Cherries
1.0	Cheddar cheese	0.4	Summer squash
1.0	Strawberry	0.3	Papaya
1.0	Asparagus	0.3	Celery
0.9	Blackberries	0.3	Cottage cheese
0.8	Red cabbage	0.3	Apple
0.8	Pumpkin		

Copper

Milligrams (mg) per 100 grams edible portion
(100 grams = 3½ oz.)

13.7	Oysters	0.5	Sunflower oil
2.3	Brazil nuts	0.4	Butter
2.1	Soy lecithin	0.4	Rye grain
1.4	Almonds	0.4	Pork loin
1.3	Hazelnuts	0.4	Barley
1.3	Walnuts	0.4	Gelatin
1.3	Pecans	0.3	Shrimp
1.2	Split peas, dry	0.3	Olive oil
1.1	Beef liver	0.3	Clams
0.8	Buckwheat	0.3	Carrot
0.8	Peanuts	0.3	Coconut
0.7	Cod liver oil	0.3	Garlic
0.7	Lamb chops	0.2	Millet

0.2	Whole wheat	0.2	Molasses
0.2	Chicken	0.2	Turnips
0.2	Eggs	0.1	Green peas
0.2	Corn oil	0.1	Papaya
0.2	Ginger root	0.1	Apple

Black pepper, thyme, paprika, bay leaves, and active dry yeast are also high in copper.

Manganese

Milligrams (mg) per 100 grams edible portion
(100 grams = 3½ oz.)

3.5	Pecans	0.13	Swiss cheese
2.8	Brazil nuts	0.13	Corn
2.5	Almonds	0.11	Cabbage
1.8	Barley	0.10	Peach
1.3	Rye	0.09	Butter
1.3	Buckwheat	0.06	Tangerine
1.3	Split peas, dry	0.06	Peas
1.1	Whole wheat	0.05	Eggs
0.8	Walnuts	0.04	Beets
0.8	Fresh spinach	0.04	Coconut
0.7	Peanuts	0.03	Apple
0.6	Oats	0.03	Orange
0.5	Raisins	0.03	Pear
0.5	Turnip greens	0.03	Lamb chops
0.5	Rhubarb	0.03	Pork chops
0.4	Beet greens	0.03	Cantaloupe
0.3	Brussels sprouts	0.03	Tomato
0.3	Oatmeal	0.02	Whole milk
0.2	Cornmeal	0.02	Chicken breasts
0.2	Millet	0.02	Green beans
0.10	Gorgonzola cheese	0.02	Apricot
0.16	Carrots	0.01	Beef liver
0.15	Broccoli	0.01	Scallops
0.14	Brown rice	0.01	Halibut
0.14	Whole wheat bread	0.01	Cucumber

Cloves, ginger, thyme, bay leaves, and tea are also high in manganese.

Zinc

Milligrams (mg) per 100 grams edible portion
(100 grams = 3½ oz.)

148.7	Fresh oysters	1.6	Green peas
6.8	Ginger root	1.5	Shrimp
5.6	Ground round steak	1.2	Turnips
5.3	Lamb chops	0.9	Parsley
4.5	Pecans	0.9	Potatoes
4.2	Split peas, dry	0.6	Garlic
4.2	Brazil nuts	0.5	Carrots
3.9	Beef liver	0.5	Whole wheat
3.5	Nonfat dry milk		bread
3.5	Egg yolk	0.4	Black beans
3.2	Whole wheat	0.4	Raw milk
3.2	Rye	0.4	Pork chop
3.2	Oats	0.4	Corn
3.2	Peanuts	0.3	Grape juice
3.1	Lima beans	0.3	Olive oil
3.1	Soy lecithin	0.3	Cauliflower
3.1	Almonds	0.2	Spinach
3.0	Walnuts	0.2	Cabbage
2.9	Sardines	0.2	Lentils
2.6	Chicken	0.2	Butter
2.5	Buckwheat	0.2	Lettuce
2.4	Hazel nuts	0.1	Cucumber
1.9	Clams	0.1	Yams
1.7	Anchovies	0.1	Tangerine
1.7	Tuna	0.1	String beans
1.7	Haddock		

Black pepper, paprika, mustard, chili powder, thyme,
and cinnamon are also high in zinc.

Chromium

Micrograms (mcg) per 100 grams edible portion
(100 grams = 3½ oz.)

112	Brewer's yeast*	55	Calf's liver*
57	Beef round	42	Whole wheat bread*

38	Wheat bran	10	Banana
30	Rye bread	10	Spinach
30	Fresh chili	10	Pork chop
26	Oysters	9	Carrots
24	Potatoes	8	Navy beans, dry
23	Wheat germ	7	Shrimp
19	Green pepper	7	Lettuce
16	Hen's eggs	5	Orange
15	Chicken	5	Lobster tail
14	Apple	5	Blueberries
13	Butter	4	Green beans
13	Parsnips	4	Cabbage
12	Cornmeal	4	Mushrooms
12	Lamb chop	3	Beer
11	Scallops	3	Strawberries
11	Swiss cheese	1	Milk

NOTE: The above values show total chromium content of these foods and do not indicate the amount which may biologically be active as the Glucose tolerance factor (GTF). Those foods marked with an * are high in GTF.

Selenium

Micrograms (mcg) per 100 grams edible portion
(100 grams = 3½ oz.)

144	Butter	51	King crab
141	Smoked herring	49	Oysters
123	Smelts	48	Milk
111	Wheat germ	43	Cod
103	Brazil nuts	39	Brown rice
89	Apple cider vinegar	34	Top round steak
77	Scallops	30	Lamb
66	Barley	27	Turnips
66	Whole wheat bread	26	Molasses
65	Lobster	25	Garlic
63	Bran	24	Barley
59	Shrimps	19	Orange juice
57	Red swiss chard	19	Gelatin
56	Oats	19	Beer
55	Clams	18	Beef liver

18	Lamb chop	3	Pecans
18	Egg yolk	2	Hazelnuts
12	Mushrooms	2	Almonds
12	Chicken	2	Green beans
10	Swiss cheese	2	Kidney beans
5	Cottage cheese	2	Onion
5	Wine	2	Carrots
4	Radishes	2	Cabbage
4	Grape juice	1	Orange

Iodine

Micrograms (mcg) per 100 grams edible portion
(100 grams = 3½ oz.)

90	Clams	11	Cheddar cheese
65	Shrimp	10	Pork
62	Haddock	10	Lettuce
56	Halibut	9	Spinach
50	Oysters	9	Green peppers
50	Salmon	9	Butter
37	Sardines, canned	7	Milk
19	Beef liver	6	Cream
16	Pineapple	6	Cottage cheese
16	Tuna, canned	6	Beef
14	Eggs	3	Lamb
11	Peanuts	3	Raisins
11	Whole wheat bread		

Nickel

Micrograms (mcg) per 100 grams edible portion
(100 grams = 3½ oz.)

700	Soybeans, dry	153	Green beans
500	Beans, dry	150	Oats
410	Soyflour	132	Walnuts
310	Lentils	122	Hazelnuts
250	Split peas	100	Buckwheat
175	Green peas	90	Barley

90	Corn	16	Beef
90	Parsley	16	Apricots
38	Whole wheat	16	Oranges
35	Spinach	15	Cheese
30	Fish	15	Watermelon
27	Cucumber	14	Lettuce
26	Liver	13	Apples
25	Rye bread	12	Whole wheat bread
25	Pork	12	Beets
25	Carrots	12	Pears
24	Eggs	8	Grapes
22	Cabbage	8	Radishes
20	Tomatoes	6	Pine nuts
20	Onions	6	Lamb
18	Potatoes	3	Milk

Molybdenum

Micrograms (mcg) per 100 grams edible portion
(100 grams = 3½ oz.)

155	Lentils	31	Cottage cheese
135	Beef liver	30	Beef
130	Split peas	30	Potatoes
120	Cauliflower	25	Onions
110	Green peas	25	Peanuts
109	Brewer's yeast	25	Coconut
100	Wheat germ	25	Pork
100	Spinach	24	Lamb
77	Beef kidney	21	Green beans
75	Brown rice	19	Crab
70	Garlic	19	Molasses
60	Oats	16	Cantaloupe
53	Eggs	14	Apricots
50	Rye bread	10	Raisins
45	Corn	10	Butter
42	Barley	7	Strawberries
40	Fish	5	Carrots
36	Whole wheat	5	Cabbage
32	Whole wheat bread	3	Whole milk
32	Chicken	1	Goat's milk

Vanadium

Micrograms (mcg) per 100 grams edible portion
(100 grams = 3½ oz.)

100	Buckwheat	10	Cabbage
80	Parsley	10	Garlic
70	Soybeans	6	Tomatoes
64	Safflower oil	5	Radishes
42	Eggs	5	Onions
41	Sunflower seed oil	5	Whole wheat
35	Oats	4	Lobster
30	Olive oil	4	Beets
15	Sunflower seeds	3	Apples
15	Corn	2	Plums
14	Green beans	2	Lettuce
11	Peanut oil	2	Millet
10	Carrots		

Other Aspects of Good Nutrition

Good nutrition must take into account four main principles:

1. Avoid all food artifacts.
2. Avoid foods to which there is an existing allergy.
3. Eat in such a way as to minimize the response to these allergenic foods to prevent the creation of new allergies.
4. Eat food that is palatable and follow a daily eating pattern which you find most comfortable.

We have already told of the harmful effect of consuming food artifacts. Obviously, the degree of harm depends upon the quantity of artifacts eaten. When rats are fed nutritious food to which is added more and more sugar, the degree of harmfulness, as measured by growth, is even greater. The rate of growth diminishes as the amount of sugar added goes up. The same rule applies to food artifacts.

Without question, the less food artifacts you use, the less harm you do your body.

We suggest that the proportion of food artifact be brought down as much as possible. At least reduce it to 20 percent of the total caloric intake. This means that all the calories provided by junk (sugar, white flour, etc.) should not exceed about 400 calories per day—a diet that will greatly increase the amount of food fiber. If there is still a problem with constipation (less than two bowel movements a day), even with the extra fiber, you should increase the fiber intake by adding bran, alfalfa tablets or any other high fiber food. Remember, foods adulterated by flavors, colors and any other chemicals that have not been shown to be safe are also food artifacts.

Single and multiple food allergies are exceedingly common, something an experienced clinical ecologist can spot immediately. Adults who have bags under their eyes which vary in color from normal flesh tones to dark, almost black, show they are allergic people. Some people have large half moons under their eyes, and even children can be affected. Usually allergy-prone people have some puffiness under the eyes. These surface blemishes are commonly ascribed to fatigue and lack of sleep. While fatigue does intensify the eye circles, it is not the true cause.

You should suspect two classes of foods (and food artifacts) as being allergens. These are the staple foods and artifacts which are eaten nearly every day, such as cereals, dairy products, sugar, and foods (and/or artifacts) which you dislike, or of which you are inordinately fond. A dislike for foods may have arisen years before from unpleasant reactions to them. The reason for the dislike may have been forgotten, but not the dislike. These foods present no problem since they are not eaten. If, however, they are introduced into the diet again for special reasons, they may make you ill.

This kind of reaction has happened with a small proportion of patients placed on a hypoglycemic diet by their physicians, or who have on their own adopted it. For example, in order to follow the rigorous diet which calls for frequent eating of high protein foods, they have had to increase their milk intake when previously they had avoided milk. After going on the hypoglycemic diet, they felt much better for many months, but eventually became ill again, experiencing depression and anxiety. This coincided with the reappearance of a milk allergy, an allergy linked to a past dislike of the milk.

One of our patients obeyed the rules of the hypoglycemic diet by eating a beef steak with each meal. He became more and more distressed until an allergist found he was allergic to beef. As soon as he eliminated beef from his eating program, he recovered.

Food or artifacts of which one is extremely fond should be looked upon with suspicion. The individual may be addicted to them based upon a chronic allergy. We have seen patients consume forty cups of coffee and sugar each day, 120 ounces of soft drink, a loaf or more of white bread or twelve glasses of milk.

To learn about your allergic addiction, it might be a good idea to make a list of all the foods you would not dream of doing without, and avoiding them for about four weeks. You will be surprised how much better you will feel once you've gone through the two week withdrawal period. This may be very intense, but it is not quite as extreme as "cold turkey" withdrawal from heroin or morphine.

While appearing contradictory to the rule we have just discussed, our advice is to eat only palatable foods. Before we were discussing not palatability, but inordinate longing or craving for certain foods. Palatability is food enjoyment. It is important to enjoy what is eaten, not only for the pleasure derived from it, but because it improves the ability of our digestive tract to digest and assimilate food.

Palatability served us well as long as we had only whole food. It was only after food artifacts came in that our palate became perverted. But we cannot depend on taste;

we should use our intelligence to select nutritious foods. It is surprising how soon we develop a liking for whole natural foods again. Many people who have scoffed at whole wheat bread as animal fodder have been amazed at how tasty it became after they stopped eating white bread. What was formerly a delicious artifact now becomes a pallid, gooey substance—consumed with discomfort.

If the above suggestions are followed, the ravages of senility will be held in abeyance for much longer periods. It is even possible that people who follow these practices all their lives may require no, or very few, nutrient supplements.

There is another important advantage to following a whole food only, allergy free, palatable diet. It will decrease the damage which will ensue if there should be a stroke or a cardiac arrest. Dr. R. E. Myers, Chief of the Laboratory of Perinatal Physiology, National Institute of Neurological and Communicative Disorders and Stroke in Bethesda, Maryland, reported at the Second Joint Stroke Conference in Miami (1977), that the real cause of damage to the brain during stoppage of circulation was due to the accumulation of lactic acid in the brain. This depended upon the amount of glucose found in the brain immediately prior to the stoppage. We have cited this study by Meyers before, but its importance causes us to emphasize it again.

He has found that monkeys starved for twenty-four hours before circulatory arrest was produced, could withstand up to twenty-four minutes before minimal neurological findings were found. In humans, it is generally accepted that four to six minutes of stoppage of blood to the brain produces irreversible brain damage.

If animals deprived of food were infused with glucose immediately before the circulatory arrest, they suffered severe and permanent brain damage after fourteen minutes. Myers found that when glucose was present, there was much more lactic acid in the brain. Normal lactate levels are 3 micromoles per gram of tissue. After ten minutes of circulatory arrest in food-deprived monkeys, lactate increased to 11 micromoles; when they were given a glucose infusion, it went up to 30 micromoles.

The work by Dr. Myers suggests that the amount of brain damage following circulatory arrest will depend upon the amount of sugar in the blood. If a patient is receiving an infusion of 5 percent glucose in saline as is commonly given in a hospital, a circulatory arrest is more apt to cause severe brain damage. For this reason, as well as others, glucose infusions should be used with great care and administered very slowly.

But there is another, perhaps even more important matter. People who follow the basic rules of good nutrition are much less apt to have elevated blood sugar levels after meals. A person who has been on food artifacts for years will suffer elevated blood sugar levels after meals. If his stroke or circulatory arrest should come on after a meal, he will be like the monkey infused with glucose, much more apt to have brain damage and less able to withstand a long period of circulatory arrest.[2]

The frequency of eating remains an individual matter. When no allergies are present, your personal preference is an adequate guide. Three meals a day seems best for most people, but some may get along well on two or even one. Others will be more comfortable with five or six smaller meals each day. When hypoglycemia is present and it is impossible to eliminate foods that cause an allergy, more frequent feeding may be the best.

The importance of good nutrition must be emphasized. Many people feel that what they have been eating for so many years could not be harmful to them. They are more apt to change their view if they accept the idea that food artifacts made them ill.

Many people want to eat well and know what they should eat, but have a deficiency in their sense of taste and smell. This may be due to a lack of zinc. We have seen several patients who could not taste food properly and found their food to be unappetizing. It required a heroic effort on their part to eat what they knew they must eat. After several months of zinc supplementation, their sense of taste and smell became normal.

The best advice on nutrition will not be heeded if there are anatomical or physiological factors which make it impossible to follow this advice. All these factors should be determined. Even fatigue may lead to malnutrition from starvation.

Several years ago, I was asked to see an elderly patient on the medical ward because he would not eat and was starving to death. When I first saw him, he weighed under eighty pounds. I learned from his chart that a few months before he had been suspected of having cancer of the stomach. He had suffered from an ulcer-type pain and had been losing weight rapidly. When his stomach was examined during surgery, a suspicious thickening was found, and the stomach was removed. Later it was found the lesion was not cancer. His post surgical recovery was poor, but after a while, he was discharged anyway. A few weeks later, he was returned as an emergency because of his being unable to eat and his suffering continuous weight loss.

In the hospital, in spite of intravenous transfusions and good care, the man continued to lose weight. When I saw him, we spoke together very quietly, and I discovered that he was normally hungry, but was too weak to feed himself. When he did get some food down, the poor fellow was so exhausted, most of it came up. I also discovered that he could retain fluids but not solid food. It was clear that he was too weak to eat or to retain his food.

I immediately started him on a milk preparation which was fortified with milk powder, and contained banana and raw eggs. The nursing staff fed him one ounce of this mixture each hour. Nicotinic acid, ascorbic acid and a few other vitamins were added to his intravenous fluid. In a few days, the man was able to sit up and feed himself.

Within a few weeks, he went on to solid food and for a while gained one pound each day. He was discharged a few weeks later on a sugar-free, high-protein diet that required frequent meals, and has remained well.

The medical intern on the case illustrates the nutritional ignorance of most recent medical graduates. After I had written my hospital orders, I received an irate phone call from the intern indicating his worry and concern. I had ordered a diet free of sugar. He reminded me on the phone that we had to restore some weight to the patient, and he could not see how a sugar-free diet could do so. He erroneously thought sugar was needed for weight gain. Fortunately for the patient, his surgeon accepted my advice and not that of the intern. I tried to explain to the new young physician, but he was too irate and hostile to listen. He never did call back after the patient recovered, his patient having gained all the weight he required.

References for Chapter Eight

1. Leisner, Pat. He slept through part of his "life." *The Advocate*, September 28, 1978.

2. Myers, R. E. Lactic acid accumulation as a cause of brain edema and cerebral necrosis resulting from oxygen deprivation. *Advances in Perinatal Neurology*. Ed. Korobkin, R. and Guilleminault, C. New York: Spedium Publishing, 1977.

9

TURN BACK THE YEARS
WITH EXERCISE

---

*I keep myself in puffect shape. I get lots of exercise—in
my own way—and I walk every day. . . . Knolls, you
know, small knolls, they're very good for walking. Build
up your muscles, going up and down the knolls.*

> —Mae West, at 61, pronouncing her-
> self in "puffect" health, news sum-
> maries of November 1, 1954. (Mae
> West is still acting in movies today
> and recently starred as a Sex God-
> dess.)

Physical Fitness Promotes Longevity

RAISED ON A FARM in Canada's Saskatchewan province
where her German parents had a large family, little Hulda
Crooks now runs three miles every day. She has climbed
14,494-foot Mount Whitney, the highest point in the
contiguous forty-eight states of the United States, seventeen
times since she first challenged the mountain in 1962—at
age sixty-six. Today, Mrs. Crooks is a jogging, hiking,
mountain-climbing great-grandmother of eighty-three.

Since starting to hike Mount Whitney, she has backpacked
the 212-mile John Muir Trail in five summer segments,
descended to the bottom of the Grand Canyon and crossed
the Sierra mountains eighty miles from west to east.

In 1978, Mrs. Crooks ran in the Orange Grove Marathon
held in Loma Linda, California, completing the quarter-

marathon of six and one-half miles in 1 hour, 28 minutes and 55 seconds. Later, that same year, the spry great-grandma set a world standard for the eighty to eighty-five age group in the Senior Olympics staged at Irvine, California.

At 5-foot-1, 115 pounds, this physical fitness enthusiast is in hardy good health that sometimes surprises even her. She keeps herself fit by following a lactovegetarian diet, an austere lifestyle, maintenance of a sense of mission to spread the message of having healthy habits, and continuous movement. She says, "Exercise you enjoy does you more good than exercise that you do because you think you have to do it. You say, "I'm going to do this. I have to do it. I'm going to do it if it kills me." And maybe it will if you do it that way."[1]

An enjoyable physical fitness program can be started at any age and at any level of fitness. And it's an important program to follow faithfully because physical fitness promotes longevity.

Being physically fit means:

1. You are not overweight or overly bulky. Very little of the body's bulk should come from the fat tissues.
2. Your muscles, bones and cardiovascular system remain in tone.
3. You feel more relaxed, active and not fatigued, except when it's appropriate to be fatigued.

The result of being physically fit is improved health, one of the best anti-aging actions to turn back the years. The process of becoming and remaining fit is primarily one of using your body by exercise or work. There is no set form of exercise, although some are more accessible than others. The main thing is to keep the body moving. Where many people spend fortunes trying to ward off the ravages of age with such surface improvements as makeup, hair dyes, toupees, face lifts and smart clothes, in reality it's exercise that does the best job. You can delay or reverse many of the deteriorating effects of aging through regular exercise.

What Kind of Exercise Program to Begin?

Machines that are used steadily break down from wear and tear. Not so the human body; it improves its functions by working. Exercise maintains the flexibility of the joints, improves blood circulation, increases breathing ability, and builds up the strength of muscles necessary to keep the spine in an upright position. It keeps in tune the harmony of all moving parts working together. Most of all, exercise helps the heart stay in good shape, and we'll have more to say later about the benefits of keeping physically fit.

Illness might impose some limitations on the normal daily activities and the regular "work out" your body gets even without engaging in a special exercise program. But there are ways around illness restrictions, too. Exercises are designed to make an elderly person feel less disabled.

Elderly people may have problems with balance, with lower reflex reaction time and with some osteoporosis. This only means they have to start slowly, but the end result can be equally valuable. No age should be considered a bar to improving one's physical fitness.

An overweight person may requir a longer time to reach the same level of fitness as a person of normal weight, but once weight begins to decrease, this handicap decreases correspondingly, as well. Being overweight means that bones are under greater stress, muscles have to work harder and the cardiovascular system has a greater burden. The overweight person shouldn't conclude that there is no point starting on an exercise program until weight is normal. Rather, begin right away and you will find that the program increases weight loss by increasing the consumption of adipose tissue for energy. The program will also decrease the appetite for excess food.

An older person already in a fairly healthy state can start a more strenuous program and expect to reach his goal more quickly. However, it is important to be realistic about your condition. Too many people grossly overestimate their own level of fitness. This can be determined by a personal test of walking fast, jogging, running or swimming to see how you become tired, pant and develop rapid heartbeat. If there is any question about your fitness to do these simple tests, then a special fitness test from a reliable expert in the field should be obtained.

Take note that exercise and overexertion are two different things. Overexertion is bad not only for the elderly, but the young don't fare so well with it either. The purpose of any exercise is to get rid of muscle pain, not to increase it; to create relaxation, not anxiety; to train the lungs, not to exhaust them; to improve circulation, not to tax the heart. Therefore, in answer to the question: What kind of exercise program should I begin? Follow these ground rules:

● Do your exercises daily, preferably at the same time each day. It is a matter of building up your capabilities, not putting them to a test.

● Exercises are best done two times a day: on arising in the morning and before going to sleep for the night. The morning exercises can begin while still in bed with prone position movements. They go along well with "morning stretching" to take the stiffness out of the joints and the sleepiness out of the muscles. The evening exercises will put a little fatigue into the muscles which enhances relaxation and helps set the stage for a restful sleep.

● Don't rush your efforts. Set no time limits and just follow your own comfortable pace—feeling *comfortable* while exercising is the key.

● Set yourself a range of motions that can be accomplished in a range of minutes. You may allow yourself 15 minutes to an hour to do your bit.

● A little heart pounding and panting after an exercise is

normal as long as it doesn't continue for longer than a couple of minutes following the exercise.

● Start out with a level and duration of exercise that causes just a moderate fatigue. This is the level to pursue patiently. After weeks and months, the amount and variety of exercises will gradually increase as you adapt to the steady pursuit of fitness. This principle of gradualness applies whether you are following one exercise or a combination. A combination is preferred so that all the musculature is made to work. If this procedure is not followed, you can expect to suffer from strains, sprains or swellings. A beginning walker or jogger who starts too enthusiastically may have sore, swollen ankles or knees. It is necessary to start slowly to allow the bones, ligaments and muscles proper time to build up their strength. From steady and gradual movement, weakened or osteoporotic bones will calcify and areas of stress will be reinforced. Ligaments will toughen and muscles will finally firm up.

● Always engage in a warming up period. This greatly diminishes the chance of pulling a muscle or ligament. Warming up is simple; merely pursue the exercise at a slow pace and gradually increase the tempo. When you are breathing easily, slightly more rapidly, and muscles feel warmer, increase the intensity of the exercise until the desirable fatigue stage is reached for that day. If walking, start slowly and gradually increase the pace until eventually the walk is as fast as possible. It would be prudent to walk for a long time before jogging and to jog for a long time before running.

Among the attitudes toward becoming fit are the two extremes: being so fearful you don't start; or being so overly confident you do great damage to yourself from over-zealous exercising. The first group of people won't be harmed by the exercise since it will never be started, but they won't benefit from a fitness program either. The second group must be cautioned not to begin too precipitously, and this applies even to those who have already been very fit and are familiar with fitness programs. They must be just as careful as a novice, but it is likely they will be able to accelerate their program. It is a process of reconditioning which can be done with maximum advantage and little discomfort.

Types of Exercise to Do

We won't describe any exercises in detail as these are available in a large number of useful books or can be obtained in a variety of fitness programs which are available. Exercising objectives should be to develop a good but not too bulky musculature; to have an efficient pulmonary-heart system which responds rapidly to increased demand and works efficiently at rest or work; to keep your bones dense, properly calcified and reinforced at the stress points; and finally, to retain your sense of balance and orientation with respect to gravity and space.

To develop, muscles must be considered as functional groups, each requiring its own particular type of exercise. Let us make some exercise recommendations for conditioning different parts of the body:

(a) *The legs*—Walking, jogging, running, swimming, bicycling.
(b) *The torso muscles—front*—This area involves any exercise which tightens the abdominal muscles against some tension. One example is to start from a position lying on your back with arms on chest or behind head and sitting up keeping knees rigid. We suggest a target of X situps, X equalling the age of the individual. Remember, each person approaches this target very slowly. There are a number of useful twisting and rotation exercises for the hip and side muscles.
(c) *The torso muscles—back*—The back muscles have the job of holding our heads up and keeping us erect. They

are potentially the strongest muscles in the body and when not working right—too tense or too flaccid—they may give a lot of pain. Low back pain is a common affliction. All back exercises consist in bending or arching the back backwards. A useful exercise is from the prone position on the floor (lying on one's stomach) to elevate the trunk with both hands on the floor. The back is arched more and more. This exercise also strengthens the arm muscles.

(d) *Arm and shoulder muscles*—Swimming and push ups are the best forms of exercise for arms. Push ups also strengthen back and abdominal muscles. Bulging biceps are not necessarily the best criteria of healthy arm muscles.

(e) *Neck muscles*—Simple rotation of the head will help. Attempt to make the largest possible circle in the air with the tip of the nose. This is done both clockwise and counter clockwise.

We have not described exercises which require any gadgets such as rowing machines, exercise bicycles, trampolines, bars, swings and so forth—not because they are not helpful, but because they are not available for the majority of people. We have drawn attention only to those forms of exercise which require a floor, a walking surface (beach, road, street) and you, plus a mat to lie on. We also have avoided referring to unnatural exercises. A natural exercise is one which has developed during evolution; as an extreme example, dragging a weight by one's teeth is not a natural exercise.

(f) *Bone exercises*—Bones bear weight and are attached to muscles. They are as light as nature can make them consistent with the necessary strength and rigidity. To make them light, they are hollow and to make them strong, they contain trabeculae. *Trabeculae* are reinforced tissue sections which buttress the bone in areas most exposed to stress and strain. The main result of disuse is loss of calcium—osteoporosis. There are no specific exercises for bone strength. The groups of exercises we've already described will also help keep bones fit, but the best are exercises like walking, jogging, running and swimming.

(g) *Balance*—Balance is learned and retained by exercises involving balance. There are a large variety. They include assuming various positions from standing on one's foot to standing on one's head. The latter requires a good deal of fitness and muscular development and elderly people who can't do this should not feel they have failed to become fit.

Health and physical fitness are both the result of a way of life which must include personal hygiene, nutrition, as described in this book, supplements of vitamins and minerals when needed—in optimum amounts—a continual program of exercise and activity which involves all the elements of movement, muscle, bone and balance. Using just one of these components alone will not result in health. We define health as the optimum possible feeling of well-being in a person who is not ill by any medical standard. We do not suggest that this feeling will lead to happiness, but it will certainly make it more probable that the individual is happy, contented or both.

There is no direct evidence that being physically fit will prevent senility, but old people who are not senile generally tend to be more physically fit, perhaps because they are more independent and mobile. It seems a prudent hypothesis that being physically fit will decrease the rate of senility development. There is pretty good evidence that it will prevent coronaries in people who have already suffered one, and should decrease the tendency to even have the first. What is good for the heart is good for the circulation, and what is good for the circulation should be good for the brain in retaining its normal function. But a program of physical fitness which ignores good nutrition and supplements is only a partial program. Unfortunately, too many physical fitness educators and leaders do ignore good nutrition.

How Exercise Improves an Aged Body

Organic efficiency as well as muscle function are enhanced by regular exercises. The result is that an aged person will get greater physical and mental health and fitness from his program of activity.

We could make an extensive listing of the various body functions that improve in the aged body from endurance exercises like jogging, walking, swimming, and others. Instead, we will outline just a few of the more significant changes you may witness from routine training. Remember, we're talking here about a regular, gradual and progressive overload to action of the muscles. Get them moving!

The large leg muscles have more than just locomotion as their job. They also aid the total circulation by massaging the blood back to the heart. Working with the diaphragm —also a muscle—the thigh muscles and calf muscles minimize the stress put on the heart muscle by acting as auxiliary heart pumps.

If you exercise routinely—appointing the same time each day for yourself to work out—you can expect some excellent cardio-respiratory changes to take place in your aged body. First, you'll increase your vital capacity and have your lungs handling more oxygen. Your lung capillaries will pull more oxygen into the blood for spreading around to the 60 trillion cells in the body, including what's left of the 12 billion cells you started with in the brain. You'll be able to incur and repay any oxygen debt with ease. There will be more rapid gaseous exchange within the lungs.

Your chest wall will get more flexible, too, aiding respiration. The peripheral circulation far away from the central cardiovascular system will have less resistance to bringing all that good blood to the outlying cells You'll be providing more effective tissue oxygenation.

During the exercise period itself, the rate and depth of respiration increases as does the rate and force of the heart beat. However, the resting heart rate will come down and the resting blood pressure, if elevated, will also come down. Steady physical fitness procedures are known to lower high blood pressure.

Small blood vessels in the skin and muscles will function better, and the red blood cell count with its hemoglobin will increase in quantity. The result? Your skin will take on a glow and the look of aging will fade.

The heart stroke volume will increase so that more blood can be pumped with each stroke of the heart muscle. Your heart pump won't have to work so hard. There will be a lowering of the resting heart rate as well as more efficient heart function, in general.

Collateral circulation, where it is needed, will build up. In some cases, doctors have noted that patients have their occluded coronary arteries open up from a program of proper diet and exercise. Nathan Pritikin, a nutritionist who directs the Longevity Center in Santa Monica, California, has reported excellent results from his clients following a strict diet and exercise regimen.

The cortisone hormone balance of the adrenal glands will be enhanced. The adrenals themselves are conditioned and fortified also, so that more severe stress may be adequately handled by your body and brain. You won't be so easily distressed by life's stressors.

We've mentioned before that elevated blood cholesterol levels tend to go down from steady exercising, provided no saturated fats are taken. There is some evidence to show that by minimizing your animal fat intake and supplementing your diet with vitamins and minerals, you'll be adding to the benefits of physical activity.

Exercise helps to maintain an adequate supply of cortisone. This doesn't aid just the adrenals, but also reduces calcium loss. Bones don't get brittle but stay strong by your physical effort. The more you move the better.

As circulatory efficiency increases, the total organic efficiency of the body, including the kidneys, liver, lungs and gastrointestinal tract tends to go into action. You get rid of wastes more effectively. Furthermore, there will be less blood waste such as lactic acid resulting from a given amount of exercise. This minimizes fatigue as well as pain related to body movement. Also, your blood viscosity doesn't thicken, and you eliminate blood clots from developing.

In general then, regular exercise improves the use your body makes of food: improves elimination; helps digestion; lessens constipation; avoids kidney stones; and even reduces the symptoms of diabetes. You'll be preventing fatty degeneration of the heart, lungs, blood vessels and brain, which might otherwise occur, as it often does, in a sedentary person.

In short, the brief amount of time you appoint yourself to exercise daily is certainly well spent. The rewards in terms of better health and fitness will compensate you many times over for the effort spent.

References for Chapter Nine

1. Kendall, John. Eighty-two-year-old granny still jogging, hiking, climbing. *The Advocate,* December 20, 1978.

10

IS AGING REVERSAL POSSIBLE WITH GH3?

On being asked if he was tired after a performance, the ninety-three-year-old cellist, Pablo Casals, said, "Why should I be? I'm the same man I was fifty years ago."
—The New York Times, January 3, 1971

THE PROMISE of prolonged youth and the testimonials of thousands of patients have carried word of a seemingly miraculous treatment far beyond the borders of the People's Republic of Rumania. Rumania is the nation of origin of Ana Aslan, M.D., director of the National Institute of Gerontology and Geriatrics. Under her supervision, a staff of 1,000 in over 200 Rumanian clinics give treatment to reverse aging using the drug she has developed called *Gerovital H3* (GH3).

Pilgrimages by notables including French President Charles De Gaulle, U.S. President John F. Kennedy, West German Chancellor Konrad Adenauer, Chinese Chairman Mao Tse Tung and Vietnamese Chairman Ho Chi Minh, were taken to acquire injections of this youth drug. Actresses Marlene Dietrich, Lillian Gish, the Gabor sisters, and actors Charlie Chaplin and Kirk Douglas and artist Salvador Dali have made the journey. They traveled to the Otopeni Clinic just outside the ancient city of Bucharest, where Dr. Aslan does her research with GH3.

Once discovered by these celebrities, GH3 itself has

become famous and is now used in over twenty countries around the world. It is available over the counter without prescription in England, Germany, Italy and Switzerland. In the United States, the Rom-Amer Pharmaceuticals Ltd. of Las Vegas, Nevada, distributes Gerovital H3. In 1977, Nevada legalized its manufacture and sale. However, the U.S. Food and Drug Administration does not approve of its distribution in any of the other forty-nine states, and the American Medical Association concurs with this ruling.

GH3 is simply the local anesthetic procaine hydro-chloride—used by dentists and podiatrists—to which has been added buffering agents and other chemicals to create a hybrid drug (Gerovital H3). The additives have transformed this local anesthetic into a new medicine that possibly reverses the aging process. How this came about makes for an interesting story and reveals a lot more about procaine and its youth restoring properties.

Dr. Parhon Discovers Professor Aslan

Intensely interested in the problems of the aging, Dr. Constantine I. Parhon founded the Institute of Endocrinology in Bucharest, Rumania, to carry on his experiments on the functions of the endocrine glands. He published the first large scale endocrinological work in medical annals fifty years ago. For forty years, Dr. Parhon continued his experiments searching constantly for the causes of aging. This drive of Dr. Parhon's to find the reasons behind aging and perhaps arrive at a solution to slow down or retard the aging process led him to establish the Institute of Geriatrics. This Institute was founded at the request of the Rumanian government in 1951. It had become the center for the study in the advanced methods for both the treatment of the aged and retarding the signs of age.

One of Dr. Parhon's staff members at the Institute of Endocrinology was Ana Aslan, M.D. For over twenty years, this doctor had been a specialist in cardiovascular diseases.

She had been interested in the pharmacodynamical properties of procaine and the reactions of this drug on the human body. Before coming to the Institute, Dr. Aslan was a researcher in pharmacology (the science of drugs) at an experimental clinic in Timisoara, Rumania. It was here that she first began using procaine in the treatment of asthma and for circulation disorders.

During her tenure at Timisoara, she uncovered the works of Dr. Gustav Spiess. He was the first to discover that procaine had many other values besides its known anesthetic qualities. He wrote reports about his experiments about the curative powers of this drug which Prof. Aslan read. After checking this literature, she extended her treatment to include patients with arthritis and limb embolisms. Another pioneer in this work was Rene Leriche whose work went further than Dr. Spiess's.

Dr. Aslan, encouraged by these reports, adjusted their methods in her practice. She also used Leriche's method, who advocated the infiltration of 10 to 25 cc and was able to restore the affected joint or limb of her patients. These patients, often after two treatments, were able to return to work and were free of pain. This increased the uses in her practice from asthmatic patients; she used it as an anti-inflammatory agent for those suffering from bone and joint diseases.

It took a dramatic incident to convince Dr. Aslan that she should continue to concentrate her efforts on developing procaine H3 for the use of the aged. She was satisfied that it had many unknown benefits. When injecting procaine H3 into arthritic joints and other areas of pain, she noticed her patients' response was most satisfactory. Joints heretofore immobile or frozen were now mobile and flexible, almost normal. Under Dr. Parhon's guidance, she continued to experiment at the fine laboratory facilities at his Institute, working to find the drug's effectiveness on the aged. Dr. Parhon is convinced that the old age process is treatable exactly as any other disease. Dr. Aslan, with her research background, advanced his theory that old age was not only treatable as a disease but could also be retarded.

Serious Medical Research with Procaine

Gerontologists concur that as the body grows older, definite physiological changes occur. Many patients exhibit the following group of symptoms:

- Premature aging with its complex group of symptoms
- Diseases of the aged—loss of memory, energy and vitality
- Diseases of the nervous system—diminished hearing abilities, visual acuity and dulled mental functions
- Diseases of muscles and joints—rheumatism and arthritis
- Diseases of skin and allergies—baldness, psoriasis, and the old appearance of the skin, face and body
- Diseases of the cardiovascular system—angina pectoris and varicose veins
- Diseases of the gastrointestinal system—ulcers and stomach disorders.

Prof. Aslan believes that the body's inherent natural ability to replace cells lost through disease and age diminishes through the years. Procaine supplements the body's ability to regenerate the cells. She is convinced that cell regeneration is responsible for a return of youthfulness to older people.

Her experiments with mice, for the next few years, substantiated her theory that besides removing the effects of a disease, it had no side reactions. In mice that developed arthritis, the beneficial effects and their return to complete mobility was most encouraging. These successes led her to treat almost 200 patients at the Institute who exhibited a wide range of dysfunctions. Some patients were suffering from old age ailments, others from arthritis and degenerative diseases.

Initially, she used procaine in a series of injections to treat twenty-five elderly patients, whose range of ailments was from arthritis to senility; she had apparent successes. None was happier than this initial group—the blessing to obtain dramatic relief from diseases that plagued them for years was heartfelt. With the signs and symptoms of premature aging diminished, Prof. Aslan was still unsure of which factors worked for her patients. The name of her treatment—GH3—intrigued her. Could it be that the component parts of GH3 were needed and used by the body? The fact is that GH3 hydrolizes in the body releasing these factors.

After working with procaine since 1947 on an experimental basis, using it for years in the treatment of specific diseases, and making a great many clinical observations, Dr. Aslan made claims for procaine: when administered properly and in certain prescribed doses, it would not only retard the aging process but would relieve chronic ailments, diseases of old age and premature aging. This remarkable claim for a drug, known throughout the world as an anesthetic, was based on treating 20,000 patients for a period of over fifteen years. Some individual patients have been treated for as long as ten years.

This backlog of patients provided her with many questions to be resolved. When it was injected into the body, why were the actions of GH3 so different from any other product? Did the body have the ability to extract the good from the ingredients found in the product?

The Claims for Procaine Injections

Speaking for the first time before an audience composed of Western scientists and doctors in 1956, Dr. Ana Aslan astounded the medical profession with her disclosures that could revolutionize the treatment of the aged. Dr. Aslan stated that procaine can benefit victims of arthritis, arteritis (inflammation of the arteries), cerebral arteriosclerosis (hardening of the brain arteries), trophic ulcers (ulcers due to improper nutrition in a particular portion of the body), alopecia (baldness), senile Parkinsonism, loss of hearing, ringing in the ears, noises in the ears, those who do not benefit from hearing aids, loss of eyesight due to aging with blurred vision, scant vision, poor eyesight, high blood pressure, defective heart conditions, those suffering from schizophrenia, ichthyosis, senile keratosis, dermatosclerosis, psoriasis, rashes and leucoderma. The therapy, stated Dr. Aslan, repigmented existing hair, improved muscle tone, improved failing memory, improved the central activity of the nervous system, improved cardiovascular reaction to stress and increased oxygen consumption. It can restore the use of limbs to those suffering from a stroke.

Dr. Aslan found from her treatments and experiments that procaine directly affects the cerebral cortex and its dynamics, and acts on the whole nervous system. The dicephalon centers, the spinal cord, peripheral nerves and metabolic processes undergo trophic changes from the procaine treatment.

Procaine is noted to be a slow-acting drug when it is not used as an anesthetic. The first few months show little or no effect. Perhaps one of the most favorable, significant observations was that the cholesterol level of almost every patient receiving treatment was brought down to normal. Many doctors believe that cholesterol found in the arteries of people approaching old age is a prime factor in the degenerative diseases of arteriosclerosis.

Procaine activity on cholesterol and its reduction from the arterial walls may be due to its hydrotrophic action, characteristic of the chloride of para-aminobenzoic acid. Doctors are also treating this condition with higher dietary intake of magnesium, pyridoxine HCL, and increasing the levels of organic potassium and calcium. The dietary plan for retarding age symptoms simply does not produce the same results for everyone. Now with GH3 Dr. Aslan, as well as other gerontologists, was seeing new appearance, mental well-being and reduced blood pressure. In some instances, oral preparations were used with similar achievements. How pleasant and simple and wonderful to provide for those wanting this help.

Dr. Aslan summed up her talk before the Academy by saying that procaine minimizes the feeling of sickness and leads to a heightened desire and capacity for physical and mental activity.

She further stated that procaine therapy has restored the original color to grey hair. After the treatments, in some people, the roots grow in according to the natural color of their hair. People with blond heads of hair once again possess heads of natural colored hair. In certain kinds of baldness, the therapy has sometimes restored hair growth. Hearing losses have been reduced in time except in those cases where there is severe nerve cell damage. Results of European experiments show that procaine was observed to have some bearing on the course of multiple sclerosis. These experiments show it to be a potent drug in treating certain blood clots affecting blood circulation.

Dr. Aslan has tested the effects of procaine on the human body for a longer period of time than have most other medical doctors. Consequently, she has had the opportunity to observe the many results of the drug. This Rumanian physician has stated that the procaine therapy appears to have a stimulating effect on the endocrine glands; she believes this is the fundamental physiological effect of Gerovital H3 on the patients. This observation is further substantiated when procaine is injected into the blood stream; it has a direct action on the body's nervous system.

She says procaine has a strong biocatalytic action affecting not only the cells in the nervous system but on the higher centers of the brain. This action aids a patient to recover partial losses of vision and improvement in hearing. Many times after undergoing a treatment or series of injections, a patient's eyes become brighter and hearing shows marked improvement. Some authorities believe the breakdown of GH3 is responsible for many reactions unknown at this time. The rapture of having one's senses return almost to normal can be understood by all of us. The energetic person wants to retain the knowledge of his years and refuses to accept the limitation of lessened mental and physical functions.

Other Uses for the Youth Drug

The success of Dr. Aslan's procaine therapy has led her to experiment in other areas of the human body and to treat a variety of ailments. The procaine treatment has been tried, as stated above, on the nervous system, in retarding multiple sclerosis, Parkinson's disease, postapoplectic conditions, osteoporosis, vitiligo, scleroderma, psoriasis, ichthyosis, on diseases of the cardiovascular system such as angina pectoris, varicose veins and on the endocrine glands. All of the above mentioned treatments have shown a measure of success.

Dr. Aslan's claims and theories have been supported by many doctors of many countries as well as by Rumanian doctors and scientists. The noted West Berlin surgeon Erwin Gohrbandt reported dramatic improvement of multiple sclerosis with procaine injections into the sympathetic trunk, particularly into the stellate ganglion and the solar plexus. Dr. P. Braunsteiner, of Rheine, Westphalia, Germany, injected several series of this injectable in a group of elderly patients who were hard of hearing. He observed that every one of the thirty-five patients selected had increased their hearing powers. In 1950, before the Congress of Internal Medicine in Paris, Dr. M. G. Good of the Charterhouse Rheumatism Clinic in London, described his successes in treating muscular rheumatism and arthritis with intramuscular injections of procaine.

Doctor H. Warren Crow, chief of the Charterhouse Clinic, has called procaine therapy "the most valuable weapon in the treatment of the individual rheumatic patient." Professor Eichholtz of Heidelberg has conducted pharmacological research on certain diseases formerly treated with calcium. His experiments showed that diseases such as bronchial asthma, urticaria and various skin edemas respond to procaine injections. The Soviet researcher, N.K. Gorbadei, reported rapid relief from ulcer pain, normalization of the secretory and motor activity of the gastro-intestinal tract, and the disappearance of the dyspepsia following procaine therapy.

Since Dr. Aslan's revelation of the discovery of procaine for retarding the aging process, there have been over one hundred papers published on the subject. There have been at least four studies made on its use in retarding premature aging. Some doctors agree that another method must be found to simplify the giving of GH3, as many times this treatment is hindered by the numerous office visits required. While the primary method is now prevailing throughout the world, oral substitutes must be found. Doctors interested in prolonging the life span and reducing the symptoms of old age are in accord for the need of another modus operandi.

Doctors in the United States showed their interest in Gerovital H3 by conducting experiments with procaine and other combinations, developed solely for hospitals, clinics and laboratories.

A study was conducted by Luigi Bucci, senior psychiatrist at New York's Rockland State Hospital and by Dr. John C. Saunders, principal research scientist and assistant in neurology at Columbia University College of Physicians and Surgeons. The two doctors found that patients suffering from schizophrenia recovered faster when given Gerovital

H3 treatments. Dr. Bucci stated that GH3 is definitely a useful medication for the treatment of aged and psychotic patients.

Another study by Dr. Joseph Smigel, director of the Pinehaven Sanitarium in Pinewald, New Jersey, reported excellent results in seventy patients out of eighty-five. Many patients who were in the younger age group have been able to leave the institution; some are back at their jobs.

Procaine may also have some value in treating hypertension, irregular heart rhythm, angina pectoris, cardiospasm, skin inflammation, hives, and as a narcotic substitute for severe pain, including the treating of addiction.

In recent experiments by Dr. Bruno A. Marangoni, chief of medicine at Flower Hospital in New York, it was found that procaine therapy is particularly effective treating paroxysmal supraventricular tachycardia, arterial fibrillation and complete heart block. Dr. Marangoni's experiments have shown that heart diseases respond dramatically to the injections.

Many drugs are used in the practice of geriatrics to reduce hypertension. Some are highly toxic and must be given under the direct supervision or constant observation of the physician. Doctors have found that procaine, having little or no toxic reactions, simplifies their treatments. Procaine's effect on a patient's high blood pressure may show a steady decline as the treatments progress; and a normal reading of some patients has been recorded by the end of the treatment series.

The claim of Rumanian doctors that procaine injections have cut the death rate for all kinds of diseases to about one-fifth was emphatically brought home at Pinehaven Sanitarium, which was involved in a respiratory epidemic that swept Orange County, New Jersey. Many patients developed a fulmination-type pneumonia, causing death within twenty-four hours. In some cases, death occurred ten or twelve days after apparent recovery due to either a cerebral or a coronary embolus. However, of the patients that had received the procaine treatment, the death rate occurred from only 3 percent to 12 percent.

Enzymatic and Biocatalytic Actions

Procaine's effect on the body's nervous system has a direct effect on the enzymes in the body. Many noted scientists feel that the degeneration of enzymes is part of the aging process. Dr. Albert White of the Albert Einstein College of Medicine wrote a paper on the aging process in the *Journal of the American Association for the Advancement of Science*. He stated this opinion on enzymes:

> The whole gamut of enzyme chemistry seems to be involved. A gradual shift of rate and directions seems to occur in the huge complex of enzyme regulation of the internal steady state in the cells, tissues, and the organism as a whole. This alteration in enzyme activity may be the real beginning of senescence.

Another authority on enzymes and the nervous system, Dr. Ivan P. Pavlov, felt that aging was caused by damage to the nervous system, particularly the cerebral cortex. Dr. Pavlov has shown that should it be possible to influence the nervous system, a change of metabolism and enzymatic processes may be achieved.

Dr. Aslan's GH3 therapy acting on the nervous system contributes to healthful action of the cells to produce proper enzyme action, which in turn is regulated by the nervous system.

No claim has ever been made by Prof. Aslan in any of her published papers that she has made a new drug discovery. However, by using GH3 over an extended period of time and in certain prescribed doses, perhaps she has found new uses for the drug's ability to retard the aging process.

The chemical formula for procaine HCL is $C_{13}H_{20}O_2$-

N_2HCL. Its generic or chemical name is para-aminobenzoic diethylaminoethanol hydrochloride or procaine HCL. It is composed of small colorless crystals soluble in water.

Biochemists have long known that the human liver produces a specific enzyme called procainesterase, which breaks down the para-aminobenzoic diethylaminoethanol releasing para-aminobenzoic acid to the body. This may well be a clue to the possible important role played by GH3 in basic biochemical processes.

Procaine HCL is one of the few drugs that completely alters its chemical composition when injected into the body. It will be recalled that procaine is rapidly hydrolyzed in the body with the formation of p-aminobenzoic acid and diethylaminoethanol.

P-aminobenzoic acid (PABA) has strong biocatalytic action. It was first regarded as a vitamin-like substance because of its biocatalytic action on such living organisms as yeast. It will, as well as procaine, inhibit sulfanilamide activity. It is not necessarily contraindicated if cognizance is taken of this effect. PABA has been used successfully in treating rheumatism, arthritis, and senile changes of the skin and hair.

Procaine HCL's aggregate of actions is that it can exert simultaneously: analgesic, sympatholytic and vasodilating; secondarily, parasympathetic and anticontracting.

The Present Treatment Methods

It is entirely feasible that men of science may successfully construct the component part of Gerovital H3 in a tablet. Biochemists call p-aminobenzoic acid vitamin H-1. The far reaching and well known biochemical action and effects of both p-aminobenzoic acid and diethylaminoethanol have been used in oral form.

In treating the diseases and ailments that accompany the aging process, quick results cannot be expected. Procaine is a slow acting drug; it is not until the third or fourth month that beneficial effects begin to appear.

There are three treatment methods. Gerovital H3 can be taken into the human body: intramuscularly, intravenously or intra-arterially, and orally, in tablet form. Some of the methods have greater absorption than others. Intramuscular injections were received by a large majority of the Parhon Institute patients. However, it is the slower of the methods, taking a much longer time to achieve the desired results. The intravenous or intra-arterial injections will react on the patient quicker. In the case of either method, a competent doctor must perform the treatments. An oral tablet would be well received by all the people of the world as an economical substitute.

Although GH3 is non-toxic, non-habit forming, and produces no side effects, the patients at the Institute still were tested for any reaction to the drug prior to undergoing the full treatment. This should be a standard practice with any patient prior to GH3 therapy.

The patient is given a small quantity of GH3 in a subcutaneous (under the skin) injection. Should the patient's reaction to the small injection be negative, another injection of 2 ml is given intramuscularly (deep into the muscular tissue). If again the patient shows a negative reaction to the injection, the full GH3 treatment may be given in complete safety. It must be remembered that the ingredient of GH3, PABA and diethylaminoethanol, is well tolerated in the body. Many doctors use oral preparations containing either ingredient for treatment and obtain gratifying results.

The course of treatment, whether intramuscular, intravenous, or oral, as modified and perfected by Dr. Aslan, consists of one injection of 5 ml of GH3 three times a week for four weeks. As stated above, GH3 has a very slow reaction in the ailment or disease, as the inroads into the affliction are slow in developing. A second course of twelve to sixteen injections is given following a mandatory ten-day rest period. Since GH3 is non-toxic and non-habit forming, as many courses as a doctor deems necessary can be administered. However, the ten-day recuperative period must be observed. The Rumanian doctors subscribe to this schedule of injections of GH3 therapy for elderly people.

A preventive course of GH3 therapy injections given middle-aged persons for retarding the aging process is slightly different. The Rumanian method of twelve to sixteen injections is followed by one to two months' resting period; then another series of twelve to sixteen injections is given. This treatment could, and usually does, go on indefinitely to forestall the aging process.

The oral method should follow the same sequence of treatment as described above for the injection method.

The inconvenience of taking GH3 injections over a long period emphasizes the necessity of perfecting another method to provide this important and valuable treatment for more people. It would be interesting if through this other method the cost could be reduced, so that economics would not prevent people from enjoying the benefits of GH3.

The GH3 Formula Revealed

Dr. Aslan's precise formula for the GH3 injections has been clouded in an aura of mystery. When she spoke before the conference on Geriatrics in San Francisco, there were confusing reports concerning her formula. One report stated her handwriting was so illegible and her command of the English language so limited, the physicians and scientists in attendance did not understand her. The other report stated she simply refused to make her formula public. Dr. Bucci, conversing with Dr. Aslan in French, was told the formula consisted of the following ingredients: 0.3 percent potassium salt, 0.3 percent sodium salt, and 0.3 percent benzoic acid as a preservative. Dr. Aslan stated that the procaine action is greatly enhanced by the addition of these ingredients.

The GH3 injections used by Dr. Aslan in treating thousands of patients over the past ten years is a 2 percent solution of procaine, available from most pharmaceutical supply houses, with a pH factor between 3.5 and 4.0. The original GH3 substance had a pH factor of between 4.2 and 5; however, this has been reduced by modification to 3.7. A substance with a pH of 7 is neutral (neither acid nor alkaline). Below the factor of 7, the substance takes on an acid activity while above the 7 factor, it has alkaline characteristics.

Experiments have proven that if procaine's pH factor is reduced, it loses some of its anesthetic value; however, procaine's effect on the sympathetic and parasympathetic nervous system is more effective. The lower pH factor of the GH3 compound is believed to be one of the reasons there are no side effects of allergic sensitivity to most patients. Dr. Aslan has suggested that any competent doctor can administer the GH3 therapy following the procedure set forth by her in any one of the papers published on the subject. She, however, warns not to use special solutions of Gerovital H3 containing other drugs than procaine, such as adrenalin, in the GH3 treatment.

There have been many procaine preparations developed in other countries with slightly different composition. In West Germany, a combination of procaine, rutin, and vitamin B-12 is called Prokopin-G or Ruticain. In Switzerland, the solution has been called Procaine Vifor. Greece's procaine injection has been labeled Procaine Minerva. Spanish pharmaceutical houses have called the solution Trophomorina-H3. Compensol and Gericain are the trade names in Argentina. In Brazil, it is called Gerontex-H3. Ecuador doctors know the procaine solution by the name of Juventocain. The Rumanian chemical export company calls its procaine solution by the name of Gerovital-H3.

There is a solution composed of dimethylaminoethanol and para-aminobenzoic acid, folic acid, several vitamins, unsaturated fatty acids and other substances called Gerioptil. Its oral counterpart is called Gerioptil plus H3.

Good Nutrition Is Needed with GH3

Further research and study into GH3 therapy as a counteraction against the aging process has given rise to the fact that proper nutrition and mineral supplements to the GH3 injections could be beneficial. The results of extensive tests among the aged population have shown that growing old is more than a decrease in certain functions; it is also a result of biochemical imbalance. Correct nutrition and minerals, which are enzymes needed for healthy cells, help bring about a biochemical balance. This theory is supported by Cecelia Rosenfeld, M.D.

In a lecture before the Humanist Council of Southern California, Dr. Rosenfeld stated that by combining GH3 therapy with nutritional guidance, excellent results were achieved; and in many instances, patients recovered with fewer series of treatments and in less time.

Although GH3 therapy can alleviate or retard diseases of the aged, such as arthritis, arteritis, cerebral arteriosclerosis, stomach ulcers, scant or blurred eyesight, ringing in the ears, noises in the ears, hard-of-hearing, certain heart conditions, alopecia, and many other conditions, Rumanian doctors and Dr. Aslan state that GH3 treatments are not the panacea or a cure-all for the aged. American doctors also have pointed out that there are failures as well as successes with GH3 therapy. The Rumanian scientists and doctors do not claim 100 percent favorable results. There are many years of research ahead to perfect the treatment; perhaps, this means cutting down not only the length of time of the treatments but the expense factor too.

Dr. Aslan's GH3 therapy may eliminate the fear of senility and the unproductive existence of people attaining advanced age. Everyone has the right to live longer, enjoy life, view life with happiness, be free of senility, and free themselves of the tensions of aging. The aging people can overcome the fears of advancing age, dependence on their children, charity or sanitariums. The ever-increasing aged population and those nearing middle-age would take a more active and happier role in society. Cell regeneration and the regeneration of damaged tissues would retard the negative aspects of the aging process.

This could very well be the breakthrough long sought by medical science in its continuous fight against aging, and the ailments and diseases associated with advanced age that afflict the human body.

EPILOGUE

Fortunate are those who actually enjoy old age.
—Talmud: *Yebamoth*, 80 b

BY NOW, you are aware that we have not offered you the elixir of perpetual youth. We have described a new way of maintaining good health which will help most people fortunate enough not to have been hit by serious accidents or degenerative diseases such as cancer. The secret to preventing senility is to stay well until eventual death.

In our earlier book, *Orthomolecular Nutrition,* we presented a general set of guidelines for staying at a high level of wellness by good nutrition and food supplementation. Here we have focused particular attention on techniques for the aging population.

Perhaps by now, we have convinced you that health while aging is not something which can be done *for* you. It is a way of life that only you are able to adopt and follow diligently. We have not offered a pill prescription or medicines that require no effort on your part, except to remember to swallow them. Rather, you have been provided with our views and how we arrived at them. But you must begin this new way of life while you are still able to do so, for once senility begins, you may no longer have control over your own thinking. The longer you have been presenile, the less apt you are to respond to the program designed to prevent senility discussed here.

219

Our program is a combination of no junk nutrition, supplemented by vitamins and minerals in optimum quantities when needed, and combined with exercise for optimal physical fitness at any age. It is a simple daily regimen, but it does require dedication and effort. The nutrients to age without senility work well when taken as part of the routine of each day.

SUGGESTED ADDITIONAL READING

Abrahamson, E. M. and Pezet, A. W. 1971. *Body, Mind and Sugar*. New York: Jove.

Adams, Ruth and Murray, Frank. 1975. *Body, Mind and the B Vitamins*. New York: Larchmont Books.

——1975. *Megavitamin Therapy*. New York: Larchmont Books.

Airola, Paavo. 1974. *How to Get Well*. Phoenix, Arizona: Health Plus.

Altschul, A. M. 1965. *Proteins, Their Chemistry and Politics*. New York: Basic Books.

Bailey, Herbert. 1968. *Vitamin E: Your Key to a Healthy Heart*. New York: Arc Books.

Bieler, Henry G. 1973. *Food Is Your Best Medicine*. New York: Random House.

Blaine, Tom R. 1974. *Mental Health through Nutrition*. New York: Citadel Press.

——1979. *Nutrition and Your Heart.* New Canaan, Connecticut: Keats Publishing, Inc.

Bricklin, Mark. 1976. *The Practical Encyclopedia of Natural Healing.* Emmaus, Pennsylvania: Rodale Press, Inc.

Cheraskin, E., Ringsdorf, W. M. and Brecher, A. 1976. *Psycho-dietetics*. New York: Bantam Books.

Cheraskin, E., Ringsdorf, W. M. and Clark, J. W. 1977. *Diet and Disease*. New Canaan, Connecticut: Keats Publishing, Inc.

Clark, Linda. 1973. *Know Your Nutrition*. New Canaan, Connecticut: Keats Publishing, Inc.

Davis, Adelle. 1965. *Let's Get Well*. New York: New American Library.

Fredericks, Carlton. 1975. *Eating Right for You*. New York: Grosset & Dunlap.

Fredericks, Carlton and Goodman, Herman. 1976. *Low Blood Sugar and You*. New York: Constellation International.

Goodhart, Robert S. and Shils, Maurice E. 1973. *Modern Nutrition in Health and Disease*, 5th ed. Philadelphia: Lea & Febiger.

Hill, Howard E. 1976. *Introduction to Lecithin*. New York: Jove.

Hoffer, Abram and Osmond, Humphry. 1966. *How to Live with Schizophrenia*. New York: University Books.

Hoffer, Abram and Walker, Morton. 1978. *Orthomolecular Nutrition*. New Canaan, Connecticut: Keats Publishing, Inc.

Hunter, Beatrice Trum. 1973. *The Natural Foods Primer*. New York: Simon and Schuster.

——Revised edition, 1980. *Additives Book*. New Canaan, Connecticut: Keats Publishing, Inc.

Jacobson, Michael F. 1972. *Eater's Digest*. Garden City, New York: Doubleday Anchor.

Kirban, Salem. 1979. *The Getting Back to Nature Diet*. New Canaan, Conneticut: Keats Publishing, Inc.

Kirschmann, John D., Nutrition Search, Inc. 1975. *Nutrition Almanac*. New York: McGraw-Hill.

Kugler, Hans J. 1977. *Dr. Kugler's Seven Keys to a Longer Life*. New York: Fawcett.

Lappé, Frances M. 1975. *Diet for a Small Planet*. New York: Ballantine Books.

Moyer, William C. 1971. *Buying Guide for Fresh Fruits Vegetables and Nuts*, 4th ed. Fullerton, California: Blue Goose.

Newbold, H. L. 1975. *Mega-Nutrients for Your Nerves*. New York: Berkeley.

Null, Gary and Null, Steve. 1973. *The Complete Handbook of Nutrition*. New York: Dell.

Page, Melvin E. and Abrams, H. L. 1972. *Your Body Is Your Best Doctor*. New Canaan, Connecticut: Keats Publishing, Inc.

Passwater, Richard A. 1976. *Supernutrition*. New York Pocket Books.

——1978. *Cancer and Its Nutritional Therapies*. New Canaan, Connecticut: Keats Publishing, Inc.

Pauling, Linus. 1971. *Vitamin C and the Common Cold*. New York: Bantam.

Pfeiffer, Carl C. 1975. *Mental and Elemental Nutrients*. New Canaan, Connecticut: Keats Publishing, Inc.

Pinckney, Edward and Pinckney, Cathy 1973. *The Cholesterol Controversy*. Los Angeles, California: Sherbourne Press.

Rodale, J. I. 1975. *The Complete Book of Vitamins*. Emmaus, Pennsylvania: Rodale Press.

——1976. *The Complete Book of Minerals for Health*. Emmaus, Pennsylvania: Rodale Press.

Rosenberg, Harold and Feldzaman, A. N. 1975. *The Doctor's Book of Vitamin Therapy* New York. Berkeley.

Stone, Irwin. 1970. *The Healing Factor: "Vitamin C" against Disease.* New York: Grosset & Dunlap.

Taylor, Renée. 1978. *Hunza Health Secrets.* New Canaan, Connecticut: Keats Publishing Inc.

Wade, Carlson. 1975. *Hypertension and Your Diet.* New Canaan, Connecticut: Keats Publishing, Inc.

Walker, Morton. 1979. *Total Health.* New York: Everest House.
———1980. *How Not to Have a Heart Attack.* New York: Franklin Watts, Inc.
———1980. *Chelation Therapy: How to Prevent or Reverse Hardening of the Arteries.* Seal Beach, California: '76 Press.

Williams, Roger J. 1973. *Nutrition against Disease.* New York: Bantam.

Winter, Ruth. 1972. *Beware of the Food You Eat,* rev. ed. New York: New American Library.

Yudkin, John. 1972. *Sweet and Dangerous.* New York: Bantam.

INDEX